Arts Therapies and the Space Between

Edited by
Christine Lapoujade, Malcolm Ross
and Sarah Scoble

ECArTE

Other ECArTE publications:

Line Kossolapow; Sarah Scoble; Diane Waller (eds.) (2001)
Arts – Therapies – Communication, Volume I
On the Way to a Communicative European Arts Therapy
Published by LIT Verlag Munster – Berlin – Hamburg – London - Wien
ISBN 3-8258-5728-X

Line Kossolapow; Sarah Scoble; Diane Waller (eds.) (2003)
Arts – Therapies – Communication, Volume II
On the Way to a Regional European Arts Therapy
Published by LIT Verlag Munster – Berlin – Hamburg – London - Wien
ISBN 3-8258-5729-8

Line Kossolapow; Sarah Scoble (eds.) (2003)
Arts Therapy: Recognized Discipline or Soul-Graffiti?
Approaches, Applications, Evaluations
Abstract Book of the 7th European Arts Therapies Conference
Published by LIT Verlag Munster – Berlin – Hamburg – London - Wien
ISBN 3-8258-7182-7

Line Kossolapow; Sarah Scoble; Diane Waller (eds.) (2005)
Arts – Therapies – Communication, Volume III
European Arts Therapy – Different Approaches to a Unique Discipline.
Opening Regional Portals
Published by LIT Verlag Munster – Berlin – Hamburg – London - Wien
ISBN 3-8258-8935-1

Sarah Scoble (ed.) (2006)
European Arts Therapy: Grounding the Vision – to advance theory and practice
Published by UPP (University of Plymouth Press) UK
ISBN 987-1-841021-64-5

Sarah Scoble; Malcolm Ross; Christine Lapoujade (eds.) (2009)
Arts in Arts Therapies: a European Perspective
Published by UPP (University of Plymouth Press) UK
ISBN 978-1-84102-225-3

Sarah Scoble (ed.) (2011)
The Space Between: the potential for change. - European Consortium for Arts Therapies Education: Selected Proceedings of the 10th European Arts Therapies Conference, London, September 2009.
e-book, Published by UPP (University of Plymouth Press) UK.
ISBN 978-1-84102-280-2

ACKNOWLEDGEMENTS

The Editors are grateful to all those who have contributed papers to this publication and for their patience as we worked together through the editorial processes. We warmly acknowledge the editorial assistance of Matthew Gammage and thank him for his diligence and willing support over many months.

ARTS THERAPIES AND THE SPACE BETWEEN

Edited by
Christine Lapoujade, Malcolm Ross
and Sarah Scoble

UPP
University of Plymouth Press

First published in the UK in 2011 by University of Plymouth Press, Roland Levinsky Building, Drake Circus, Plymouth, Devon, PL4 8AA, United Kingdom

A catalogue record of this book is available from the British Library

Paperback ISBN 978-1-84102-289-5
Hardback ISBN 978-1-84102-290-1

Library of Congress Cataloging in Publication

Arts Therapies and the Space Between
Edited by Christine Lapoujade, Malcolm Ross and Sarah Scoble

Typeset by University of Plymouth Press in Adobe Garamond Pro 10/12pt

Printed and bound by CPI Group (UK) Ltd, Croydon, CR0 4YY

CONTENTS

INTRODUCTION
Arts Therapies and the Space Between

The arts therapies have emerged from centuries of experimentation and exploration and offer the client new opportunities to work creatively, to develop himself and to change - within a secure environment. Arts media (visual arts, dance, theatre, music, poetry) are experienced by the arts therapy client within a creative space and within the relationship between himself, the therapist and the art form. Within the framework of an inter-personal situation, repressed material can be represented by the client and handled both self-reflectively and as a direct encounter with the therapist, thereby providing opportunities for fresh understandings and the opportunity to create new connections.

Questions arise as to the specific nature of the 'space between' which might allow the possibility of making new relationships, thereby alleviating the client's difficulties, and on the implications of the concept of a 'space between' for therapeutic practice. The contributors to this book explore these issues through a range of different arts therapies. The book focuses particularly upon 'space between' client and therapist as a way of opening a wider debate about the nature of therapeutic change. The following questions characterize a key and continuing debate within the profession. What are the expectations of the clients in this special space? What are they getting from their therapy? How might arts therapists enable clients to create, develop and inhabit a 'space between': that is to say between internal and external realities, between physical and mental spaces? And how might arts processes and art forms work to open up and link these different spaces? How might an engagement in an arts therapy space create connection where there is disconnection? And how might it create new opportunities in relationships, which allow changes to occur? In what ways might different therapeutic approaches within this space influence arts therapists' processes?

The authors of the papers which constitute this publication, coming as they do from different countries, are eclectic with respect to their approaches to the theme, depending on their individual theoretical backgrounds and the special nature of their commitment, and given a particular art practice.

Thus, for J. K. Dubowski (UK), psychoanalysis has always occupied the space between consciousness and the unconscious. Images that are created through the artistic use of 'active imagination' can provide the unconscious with an opportunity to reveal significant aspects of itself, that, through interpretation, may then enter into consciousness.

Vincent Estellon (France) argues that therapy runs the risk of upsetting the symptomatic framework that upholds or supports the creative process. Healing, he proposes, is not so much a matter of eradicating the symptom, but rather of composing with one's neurosis, rendering it more creative.

David Read Johnson (USA) explores the way the perception of difference opens a space for change. As soon as difference is noted, preference follows, for if there is difference, then the whole has been split and the person is incomplete. This incompleteness arises within us as desire that informs our next action. The 'playspace' allows us to engage with difference and proximity, to learn to tolerate it, delight in it and fear it less.

In her paper, Edith Lecourt (France) develops her own, practice-based reflections on the themes 'the space between' and 'the potential for change', and comments on their place and function in the arts therapies more generally, drawing upon the writings of authors such as Winnicott, Bion, Meltzer, Bick Bollas and Anzieu.

Marián López Fdz. Cao (Spain) explores ideas around the concept of creation associated with dominance and power over others. The paper analyses some of the fundamental characteristics of creativity in the contemporary world to elicit an alternative conception linked to caring and sharing, which can become a dynamic space for art therapy.

Mimmu Rankanen's (Finland) concern is with the functions and implications that are manifested in the space between moving and touching, looking and feeling, thinking and symbolising both in undertaking the physical movement work and reflecting on the images produced in the course of therapy.

Malcolm Ross (UK) argues that there is much to be gained by conceiving of creative change in the arts as a moment of 'illumination' – rather than, as has been the more familiar case in the Western tradition, as a series of discrete, 'problem-solving' projects. He introduces his cyclical Syncretic Model based on Chinese Five Elements theory to argue his case.

The final contributor is France Schott-Billmann (France), who suggests that the dance therapist aims to restore the client's relationships with others within the transitional space of the dance. The essential rhythmical patterns of the dance are adapted to form the basis of the links: the link to oneself, to others and to the group. Memories of rhythmical games between the mother and the child are transferred in the rhythms of the dance.

Both therapy and art occur in the space of consciousness. Having said that it must be immediately apparent that there is more to be said. What, for instance, are we to say for the place of the unconscious, of what we might call unreconstructed impulse, in both these practices? And what about 'super-consciousness': the realm of divination – of creative insight, intuition and inspiration? Arranging these three notions as a continuum we locate consciousness itself as the 'space between' the unconscious and the super-conscious, as the potential space where the id and the superego cross over. Since both artist and therapist inhabit this 'space between' we have a clear rationale for the transformations we might hope for in arts therapy, namely, the creative, mutual reconciliation and adaptation of human aspiration and pretension.

The editors of this volume are delighted to be able to publish the papers selected here and have every confidence that readers will find them to be as challenging and as insightful as we have.

ECArTE Publications Committee, June 2011

Analytical Art Psychotherapy: The Marriage between Art Therapy and Analytical Psychology

Janek Dubowski

It seems to me that psychoanalysis has always occupied the space between consciousness and the unconscious and a decade has passed since Robert D. Stolorow (2000: p150) asked that we throw off "the philosophical shackles that Freud inherited from Descartes". Stolorow attempts to replace Cartesian duality (mind-body), which he points out resulted in Freud's idea of the *isolated mind*, with the idea of an *intersubjective system* that resides "at the interface of the interacting experiential worlds of patient and therapist" (Stolorow 2000: p149). Traditionally, psychotherapy (and I include art psychotherapy here) has sought to map this perceived lacuna through the use of narrative, through the so-called talking-cure. Now, we can regard the narrative itself as forming the interface between patient and therapist. Artists however have always had the ability to go beyond disembodied words and give this place tangible form. Images that are created through the use of *active imagination* can provide the unconscious with an opportunity to reveal aspects of itself – and that through interpretation, to enable these aspects to enter into consciousness. Narrative is applied in order to find meaning in what was hitherto unconscious - in other words, narrative is used in that space in-between the artist and the art therapist. Hermeneutics forms both the structure for understanding these narratives within the therapy itself and the methodology underpinning this paper. The ideas discussed come from the analysis of images and their accompanying narratives created during a series of 'workshops' during which I have explored working with the mandala with small groups of between six and twelve participants. Over the years that I have been conducting these mandala workshops I have collected well over one hundred images. For the purposes of this paper I will focus on just one image and not only that, but on a single fragment of that image, as I believe it provides a good example of *inbetweenness.*

As therapists we frequently have to position ourselves in-between. First of all there is the place in-between the client's unconscious and the therapist's consciousness. The image made by the client also occupies this space and it in turn also has the function of standing in-between the client's consciousness and his or her unconscious. The *unconscious* contains within it (or has as its core) the instincts[1]. In terms of evolutionary development (phylogeny), it is clear that consciousness arises out of a pre- or unconscious state of being. So it is with our own personal development (ontogeny) as an individual. For Freud, the relationships between these states was described in terms of the *id* (unconscious instincts), the *ego* (self) and the *super-ego* (conscious and socially determined). So, it is through the capacity for consciousness that we are able to first accept then bring under control, some of our unconscious impulses. Also associated with the unconscious, we must include at least some of the primary emotions, the mechanisms by which we can discern between elation and threat in our experience of the world. Jung makes the distinction between *thinking function* and *feeling function*[2], personified perhaps, as Logos and Psyche. *Psychology*, in a literal sense, is the study of the relationship between these two poles, the attempt to understand the Logos of Psyche. This attempt, whether under the guidance of a therapist or not, results in what we call *psychological mindedness*, the beginning of a new dialogue between the unconscious and consciousness.

The unconscious or *unknown* has many faces, psyche, soul, and spirit are terms often used in order to distinguish between the outer objective reality of the physical world (through the function of Logos) and our inner world reality. The "reality of the soul" is described by E. Neumann:

> "The reality of the soul is one of the basic and most immediate experiences of mankind; it permeates primitive man's whole view of life, naturally without his being aware that it is an inner experience. The animating principle of mana, the effect of magic, the magical efficacy of spirits, and the reality of collective ideas, dreams, and ordeals are all governed by the laws of this interior reality which modern depth psychology is trying to bring to the surface. We must not forget that the discovery of the objective, external world is a secondary phenomenon, the result of human consciousness endeavouring, with infinite labour and the help of

---

[1] Instinctual behaviour is evident in all animals and it is therefore a *pre-conscious* mechanism. Stephen Jay Gould (1977: p96), however, refers to it as *un*conscious: "Instincts are the unconscious remembrance of things learned so strongly, impressed so indelibly into memory, that the germ cells themselves are affected and pass the trait to future generations".

[2] As we often see in our clients, some who are so stuck in thinking that they seem unable to feel (*seemingly emotionally illiterate*) or those so caught up in feeling that they are no longer able to think. The work of therapy finds a definition here.

> the instruments and abstractions of modern science, to grasp the object of such, independently of the primary reality of man, which is the reality of the psyche."
>
> (Neumann 1973: pp 209-210)

So it is also this same pattern of development that we see in our own individual development from infancy towards the establishment of *self*. Our earliest experiences are of an inner-world of emotion and visceral sensation, and our initial ability to discern between inner and outer sensation is still very primitive. Only gradually do we begin to turn our attention, our focus, from the inner world to the outer and it is in forming a relationship between inner and outer that the self or ego begins to take shape.

We can see patterns and parallels between evolutionary, historical and personal development and each individual has a share in these processes. Our own personal history is also a part of a greater history, belonging first to immediate family, then extended family, community (or in some societies, tribe), then nation, etc.. We also contain within us, at the cellular level, encoded in our genetic material, the evolutionary history of our species. Some of these processes are *personal* to the individual, his or her unique history. Other aspects, such as family or tribal history are shared or as Jung stated *collective*. This distinction between *personal* and *collective* extends to the realm of the unconscious and is one of the corner stones of Jungian theory.

To return to personal development or ontology, we have seen that the process of individuation, of becoming an aware autonomous self, unfolds during infancy and childhood. Later in childhood, the development of communicative skills such as language and other non-verbal forms of communication such as art begin to unfold and it is to the development of art that we will look next.

Initially, the marks the child begins to make appear as meaningless scribbles. Next, the child begins to organise these random marks into some form of pattern, perhaps repeating the same kind of mark over and over again or combining different movements of the hand together to produce new configurations. As hand-eye co-ordination improves so the repertoire of different marks increases until the child begins to form an unusual and complicated mark that we call a circle. The discovery of the circle marks a turning point in drawing development. The circle has unusual properties in that it has an inside and an outside. Perhaps it is this simple distinction that catches the imagination of the child, reflecting and echoing the child's own experience of inner and outer worlds, of reflection and imagination, waking and dreaming, feeling and thinking. The circle also provides a gestalt: the distinction between figure and field. It stands out on the sheet of paper just as a person stands out against the landscape. As such, the circle constitutes itself the first figurative art that the child will produce – typically by placing dots for eyes on the inside and a few lines attached to the sides and bottom of the outside of the circle.

Might the artists who painted on cave walls so many thousands of years ago have gone through a similar form of development? I feel that the answer must be a definite yes, that the evolution of humankind is an evolution of consciousness and that human consciousness is marked by the evolution of language giving rise to *Logos*, or thinking function. Further, the development of channels of non-verbal communication such as art must have parallelled that of language. An understanding of symbols then, is an understanding not only of the *personal* but also of the *collective* because in the development of every individual child, we have recapitulated, the evolutionary development of everyone. The discovery of the circle that every child makes is also the discovery of the symbolic: it marks a moment in which the individual catches a first glimpse of the collective, a moment at which the unconscious and consciousness make real contact, when the inner world sees a bridge to the outer.

Another way that a distinction between inner-world (unconscious) and conscious reality is made is through primary and secondary processes. The former, as unconscious phantasy, "...does not distinguish between opposites, fails to articulate space and time as we know it, and allows all firm boundaries to melt in free chaotic mingling of forms" (Anton Ehrenzweig 1967: p.3). Ehrenzweig goes on to say,

> "Art, on the other hand, appears the embodiment of rigorous organization. So it has been assumed that art's structure is exclusively shaped by conscious and pre-conscious functions, the so-called secondary process. But this will not do."

He goes on to cite Marion Milner's Freud-Centenary Lecture on *Psychoanalysis and Art* (Milner 1958) in which she demonstrated how art reflects the inner-world just as accurately as it does the outer-world of physical reality. In a sense, this is also the point at which the profession of Art Therapy is born: a therapy with, as its central basis, an exploration of the inner-world through the making of art and the analysis of art as a bridge between the unconscious and consciousness.

On the use of circles or mandalas

Jung frequently returns to the circle as a symbol of the self and the mandala as a specific form of self-symbolism[3]. The significance of mandala images has long been recognised and used by art therapists. Whether these images are produced spontaneously (through a non-directive form of art therapy) or through invitation by the therapist they continue to provide opportunities for gaining psychological insight for our clients.

I have shown how central the discovery of the circle is to the individual

[3] In the case of "Miss X" (Jung 1959) the analysis and reproduction of a series of mandalas produced by one of his patients is provided.

development of art in early childhood and suggested that in discovering the circle the child also discovers the symbolic. For Jung, the circle or mandala features as a symbol of the unity of the 'self',

> "...which should be understood as the totality of the psyche. The self is not only the center, but also the whole circumference which embodies both conscious and unconscious; it is the center of this totality, just as the ego is the center of consciousness" (Jung 1968: p106).

Mandala symbols can be found in dreams, (Jung himself collected several hundred such dreams) and are regarded as symbols of the self. For these reasons, and through my own experience as an art therapist, I have been utilising mandalas in my work with both clients and students for some years. The rest of this paper will explore this particular technique in some detail.

I have already mentioned the importance of *psychological mindedness* and I consider that it is not until the client has achieved this satisfactorily that this technique should be attempted. A short period of engagement with more traditional art therapy, in the making and analysis of art, should, in most cases, bring the client into sufficient psychological mindedness and I have found this technique to be of particular use as a form of assessment or diagnosis during the early stages of therapy. The client should have demonstrated an ability for spontaneous art making, for allowing the quality of art materials themselves to lead in the production of forms and images. In other words, to relax conscious control and allow *things to happen*.

The initial mandala, or template, on which the client is invited to work, should be constructed by the therapist prior to the session. As the client will be invited to actually sit within the mandala it must be of sufficient size, a square sheet of paper (it should be an exact square) measuring approximately one metre by one metre. Within the square the therapist should draw a large circle with the circumference not quite meeting the edges of the square. The circle should be just large enough to contain the seated client (Fig.1).

Before being invited to sit within the mandala the client is invited to select a collection of preferred art materials and should have a full set of colours at hand (it does not matter what media the client selects, paint, crayon, pastels etc., but it should always be of the client's choice). In inviting the client to sit in the mandala s/he is also asked to place the selected materials within reach of their dominant hand. Once sat down I ask that they become aware of the two forms surrounding and containing them, first the circle, then the square. In containing and supporting them, I suggest, they might be seen as a representation of the client's 'world'.

Next, I ask that they become aware of that segment of the mandala that is situated by their dominant hand and it is in this space that I ask them to make their first mark or symbol.[4]

The instruction is: "produce a symbol that stands for you in the 'here and now' a symbol for how you are at this moment in time". In attempting to facilitate spontaneity I do not give much time for this first symbol, one or two minutes at the most. Once completed, the client is invited to contemplate how it now feels to be contained within the mandala and this first symbol before being invited to produce the second.

This is to be situated where the other non-dominant hand rests and the client is invited to "produce a symbol which is the opposite of the first symbol", again, only one or two minutes are given for this before again inviting the client to consider how it now feels to be contained within the mandala with these two opposing symbols to his or her left and right. Next, the client is asked to place their hands directly behind them and in this portion of the mandala "to produce a symbol for your past". (At this point most people have to change how they are seated in order to turn around and paint or draw). After one or two minutes, they again sit in their original position and contemplate how it now feels to be surrounded by the three symbols before being invited to produce the fourth and final initial symbol.

Now they are invited to explore the portion of the mandala that is immediately in front of them and "to produce a symbol for your future, your hopes, anticipations or fears, of the future". Following the production of this fourth symbol they again sit in the centre and time is given for them to consider how it feels to be surrounded by these for symbols, "the 'here and now', its opposite or polarity, the past behind you and the future ahead" before moving to the next stage of the session. (Fig. 2)

Initial analysis

In viewing the image together at this point there are a number of indicators that I am interested in discussing with the client, most of these initial points of focus concern composition rather than an analysis of the symbols themselves[5].

The first indicator concerns the placement of any (or sometimes all) of

[4] Jung refers to the symbol as a product of the unconscious, accordingly, it is not considered possible to 'consciously' produce a symbol. Products of consciousness are considered as 'signs'. However, the capacity that we call the 'imagination' allows for a relaxing of conscious control in order to provide the unconscious with the opportunity to express itself. Spontaneous art making can be seen as an example of 'active imagination' as described by Jung (1985: p194).

[5] The main reason for this is that later in the session (and perhaps subsequent sessions), the client will be asked to further elaborate the mandala image by exploring the relationship between the four symbols, as *products of the unconscious*, the full meaning behind the symbols is as yet un-revealed, as Jung so often said about the nature of the unconscious, "it is just that, we cannot know it" (Face to Face 1959). It is only through a more thorough analysis, which will take place later in the therapy, that the meanings behind the symbols may begin to unfold.

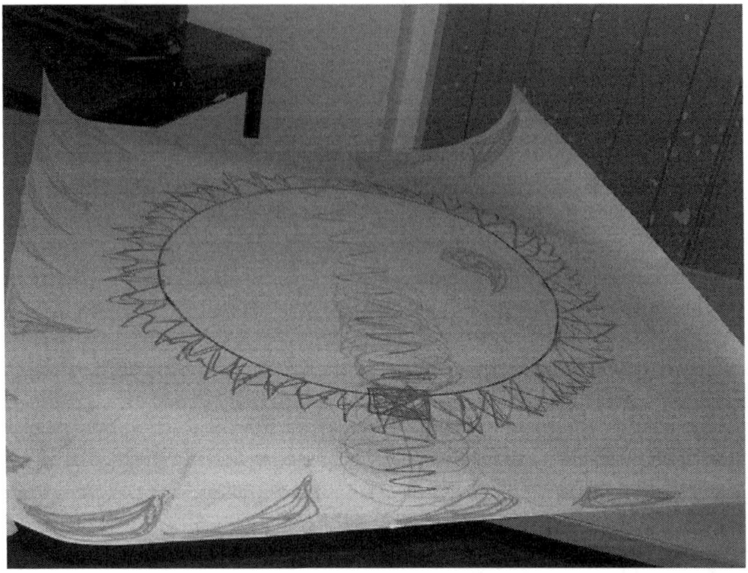

Figure 1

the four symbols in either the square (the four corners) or within the circle, or on the circumference – between the circle and the square (see Figs.2 & 3). Next, I am interested to discuss the relationship, first between axes A&B (see Fig.4) which denotes a *polarity* within the client's personality.

Sometimes this polarity concerns primary emotions, love and hate, anger and sadness for example. Or it may signify a polarity between feminine and masculine aspects, anima and animus. Frequently clients associate this axis with conscious and unconscious aspects of the self.

Finally, we will briefly discuss axes A&D (see Fig.5), the relationship between the client's past and his or her future. This initial analysis normally takes the form of the therapist simply pointing out these compositional relationships and asking the client to think about them before moving onto the next stage.

Following this initial directed sequence of the session the client is given the opportunity of working in more detail on the personal mandala, again they are urged to work spontaneously and now to explore the relationship between the four symbols, adding other symbols as they spontaneously occur.

Figure 1 shows such a mandala during an early stage in its creation. The future, represented by the orange triangle is linking to the past in the form of the grey square. The artist has been playfully exploring these two polarities first of all with the darker zig-zag line and then with colour, yellow and green predominating. Following this a grey cloud-like form passes of the past.

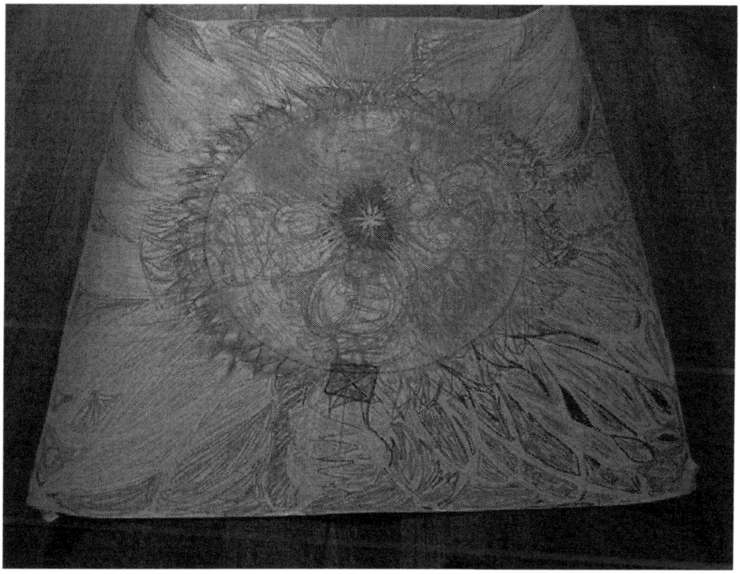

Figure 2

We should note that the initial symbols for future and past are drawn over the circle as is the first symbol for the 'here-and-now', a green square on the left, hardly visible because it is drawn in such a faint manner,. Its opposite, the red foetal form (my interpretation) is the only symbol of the four initial marks that lies within the circle rather than on it. This is left alone and it is the space between past and future that occupies the artist during this time. Following the linking of past and future the mandala circle itself is worked on with both zig-zag and wavy lines, echoing the types of mark used between past and present. Green is then used to draw large petals from the mandala circle itself, radiating to the edges of the paper. Finally, blue is used to produce the triangular forms at the edges and between the petals. This constitutes the early life of this mandala. In its execution a narrative can be seen to be emerging – whether conscious or unconscious to the artist we cannot know – and to interrupt them in their work to ask would 'break the spell' (my metaphor).

In figure 2 we can see the finished image and note how the four initial symbols have evolved. Something new has formed at the centre and everything else appears to revolve around that. The eye is drawn to it and we have to actively shift our gaze in order to note what else has changed. The past-future axis remains visibly in place but replacing the predominant zig-zag we have more of a wave. The self-axis has also been worked on and there are at least two features to note. First of all the initial green square has been considerably expanded. Secondly, its opposite, the foetal form now has three companions appearing to move from the much-expanded green square across the axis, becoming increasingly developed as they join the original symbol. The petals have been greatly worked on and it is the

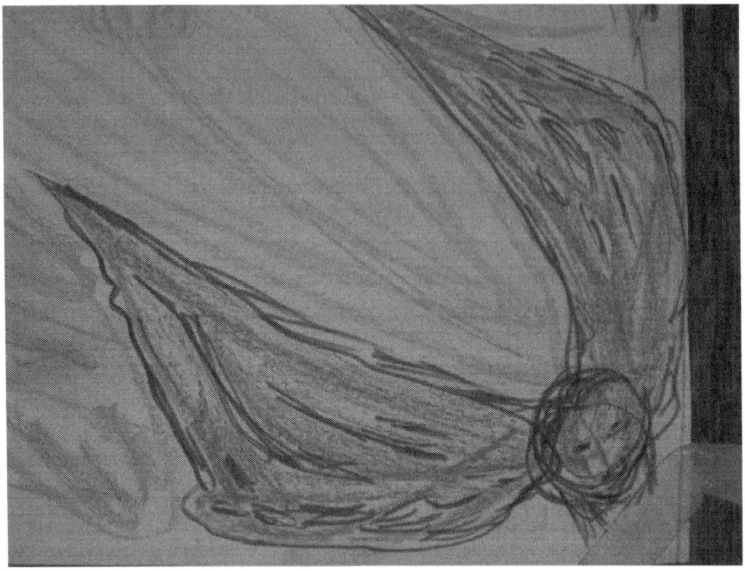

Figure 3

use of the blue at the edges of the image that triggers the creation of an unexpected and intriguing new symbol. One has to look to find it but there in the top left-hand corner of the mandala, the blue triangular forms become the wings on an angel and it is this symbol that I want to focus on – the journey or narrative of its creation, its conscious meaning (for the artist) and its unconscious content.

"The angel was facing away from me when it appeared – it started as a circle and turned into an outward looking face." These are the artist's own words: the angel "appeared", it was a product of the unconscious, a visitor from the inner-world, a messenger. She continued, expressing, perhaps, some of the message to be delivered by the angel – "I have been aware of a need to shift from my introspection and rather hypochondriac self regard. After one has acknowledged one's wounds (earlier there had been an exploration of 'the tears' in the mandala) you allow them to heal and not continually poke them. The scars do remind you of past problems at times but this is a necessary protection." Here the message is clear, dwelling on the past can be harmful and introspection can make you ill. The angel is located in the upper left-hand corner (if one regards the future to be at the top and the past at the bottom), he/she 'appears' in that part of the mandala that holds the future and he/she looks outside of the painting into the outer world of physical reality. The artist continues – "I have been aware of angels in my life since I was a very young child, but as silent beings seen out of the corner of my eye. Now I'm beginning to hear them more often. Messengers are turning up – most of them are men but the face could be either as the messenger can be both genders". Here, in regarding the gender of the angel we need to look at the archetypes of anima an animus. She states that most of the angels she encounters are male – her animus, but here it can be "both genders", but she does not say one or the other. Both suggest the angel is both anima and animus (or, arguably, it is either androgynous or a hermaphrodite). She goes on to state, "The angel is very much a symbolic instruction to watch and listen with awe and wonder at the riches of the life that flows hidden behind the fear of poverty – of not having and being enough - or the fear of being unlovable or unacceptable". These are the artist's own personal observations and we have to accept them as an honest interpretation of what has been created.

However, we must also consider the polysemic nature of all symbolic material. Unlike signs, which always point in just one direction, symbols have the capacity to hold multiple meanings – they are often considered to be 'living entities' in their own right. From this perspective we can look at a variety of meanings that potentially arise in respect to the angel. First of all, the artist does not comment on the fact that the angel is looking outwardly. That is, facing away from centre of the mandala. She does, however, later acknowledge that she is familiar with the angel motif, especially in paintings that follow the mandala tradition such as *The nine choirs of angels* from St. Hildergarde of Bingen. In this painting (now unfortunately lost, only reproductions survive) the ranks of angels all face inwardly looking towards the centre which features a blank circle, a symbol long associated with God as the circle has no beginning and no end. If we return to our mandala in the light of this, the angel looking away from the centre might be considered a *fallen angel.* In many respects our mandala conforms to classical interpretations in the centre holding the *self.* We note the light exploding from the centre – the centrality of self, and then we consider the angel again. S/he is at one of the extreme edges of the mandala, the upper left corner, located between the symbol for the non dominant here-and-now and the future and s/he is looking out and away from the rest of the painting. Not only is the angel facing away in the painting, s/he was also facing away from the artist when s/he appeared (in other words, the artist was facing the painting from the bottom rather than from the outside upper edge) when the angel appeared. So we have a symbol from the unconscious entering consciousness with a message or messages for the artist – and, in the context of therapy, for the therapist. There is a flow between consciousness and the unconscious that flows as the artist paints. This flow is a form of narrative in its own right, it forms part of the painting while staying outside of the finished painting. We need to pay as much attention to the narrative as we do to the finished image – both form part of whole. The therapy is in the flow, the narrative, the communication between inner and outer worlds of existence – coming together, bridging, become whole, becoming one.

Earlier I suggested that the making of an image forms in itself a form of *narrative,* that as the image changes, alters, parts are re-worked, others worked over, some obliterated, sometimes to be re-formed later, some covered or even destroyed – all of this is a form of narrative and the story it tells is different from the story of the finished image in many ways. For example, the making process is dynamic while the finished image is still. The dynamics of making have their own energy, direction, and emotional charge – a vertical line, for example, drawn towards the artist has a different feel, emotional charge, and meaning, from a vertical line drawn away from the artist. In the finished image, to a large extent, this dynamic is lost and we cannot tell how the vertical line was produced, away or towards – but the narrative will be so different if only we can tell. This is just one example, the order of the painting, the thickness of the paint, even the age of the brush we select, all of this can be part of the narrative of making. It always strikes me that the secondary narrative that takes place after the image is finished, when together with the artist/client, we look at it and I ask what it is about – a very different narrative is produced, lacking the dynamics and energy and emotionality I may have observed in watching the image unfold. For me, I now understand that what I call the narrative of making is actually the narrative that takes place been the unconscious and conscious mind of the artist, and the secondary narrative something that takes place between two conscious minds. We need to hold in mind and question both narratives if the full meaning of the image is to be revealed.

Postscript

2009 saw the publication of *The Red Book* by C. G. Jung. This extraordinary volume includes a number of reproductions of a series of paintings, many of which are mandalas, created by Jung himself. Perhaps this publication will rekindle an interest in the use of the mandala within therapy.

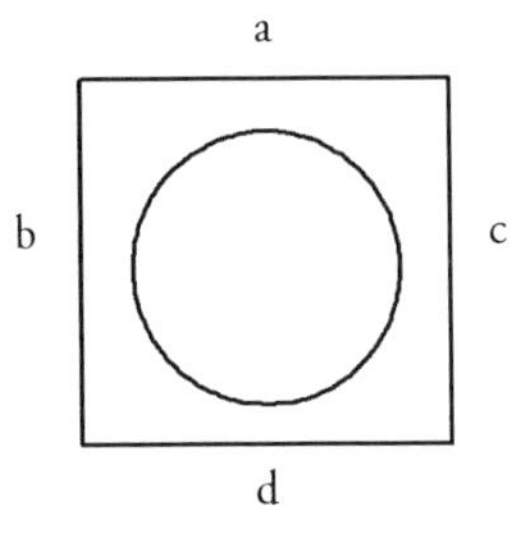

Figure 4

a Directly behind – the PAST
b Dominant hand – the HERE & NOW
c Non-dominant side – the OPPOSITE
d Directly in front – the FUTURE

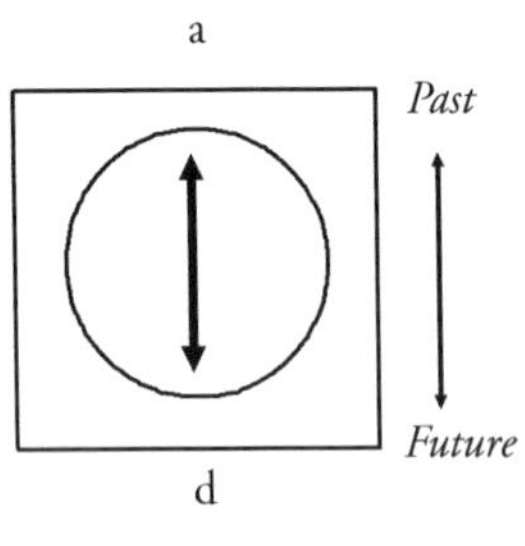

Figure 5

This axis (a – d) delineates the *relationship* between the past and the future. It provides opportunities to explore how the past affects both the here and now and our attitudes to the future. For example, how unresolved issues in the past impact on us in the here and now and how these influence our potential futures.

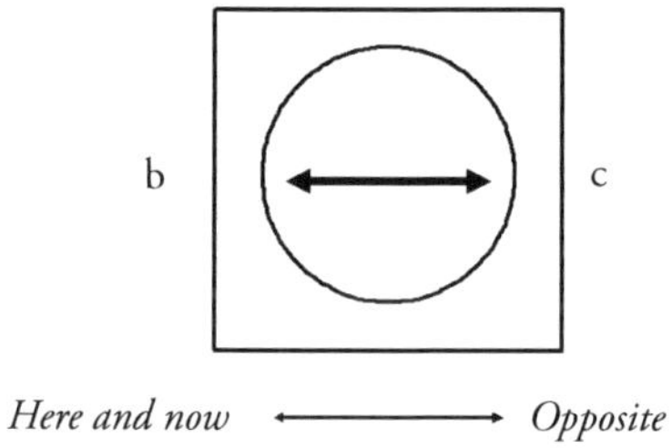

Figure 6

This axis delineates the relationship between opposite or oppositional aspects of the *Self*. It provides opportunities to explore polarities and archetypes.

References

Ehrenzweig, A. (1967) *The Hidden Order of Art*. Berkley, University of California Press.

Gould, S.J. (1977) *Ontogeny and Phylogeny*. Cambridge, Massachusetts, Harvard University Press.

Hillman, J. (1975) *Re-Visioning Psychology*. New York, Harper Colophon Books.

Jung, C.G. interviewed by John Freeman on *Face To Face*. BBC Television (1959)

Jung, C.G. (1968) *Psychology and Alchemy* in *Collected Works, Volume. 12*, 2nd edition London, Routledge.

Jung, C.G. and Kerenyi, C. (1985 – Revised Edition) *The Science of Mythology: Essays on the Myth of the Divine Child and the Mysteries of Eleusis*. London, Routledge.

Milner, M. (1958) *Psychoanalysis and Contemporary Thought*. London: Hogarth Press

Neumann, E. (1954 reprinted 1973) *The Origins and History of Consciousness*. New York, Princeton University Press

Schenk, B. (1982) The Phylogeny of Art. Aspects of the Development of Prehistoric Art. In Koch, W.A. (ed.) *Kulturund Evolution 1: Semiogenesis*. Frankfurt Verlag Peter Lang.

Stolorow, Robert D. (Spring 2000) From Isolated Minds to Experiential Worlds: An Intersubjective Space Odyssey. *American Journal of Psychotherapy*, 54 (2).

Creativity in Art and Therapy

Créativité artistique et psychothérapie

Vincent Estellon

Résumé

Dans la thérapie, la parole devient souvent l'objet d' un jeu... de cache-cache avec elle-même : un sens inattendu se fait entendre au détour d'un trébuchement de la langue, caché ou surexposé dans la logique interne d'une phrase, comme né de la capacité d'écoute de l'interlocuteur. Dans cette curieuse expérience, la parole découvre ou redécouvre sa propre ressource poétique, sa force métaphorique. Le sujet peut se surprendre à changer le sens des repères fonctionnels et utilitaires de sa propre parole mais aussi de son écoute. Le domaine du rêve, trop longtemps assigné au sommeil de la nuit, apprivoise cette parole, restée comme morte à son propre écho et lui apprend à s'entendre autrement. Par l'ouverture de ce jeu, la créativité peut être réanimé dans la parole comme dans l'écoute.

If creativity is used in both art and in therapy, it does not have the same finality and is not used to the same ends. Amongst the aims targeted by therapy, beyond that of easing the suffering of a being, helping identify key elements in their way of functioning, of freeing them from constraints or shackles, I would say that one of the signs of a successful therapy, is when something in the relationship to creativity is reanimated.

Therapy runs the risk of upsetting the symptomatic framework that upholds or supports the creative process. A pianist who came to consult me had well understood this: he didn't want to get well because in order to plunge himself into the universe of Schumann he felt the need to be acquainted with suffering, distress, exhaustion. On this level he didn't want to modify anything at the risk of no longer playing the piano. Having read a large number of psychoanalytical texts, he asked me to merely help him to understand himself better in order to better comprehend his ways of functioning and thus avoid the compulsion for repetition. What I want, he said, is not to *be well* but rather *not to repeat my mistakes*, always the same mistakes. Healing is not so much a matter of eradicating the symptom, but rather of composing with one's neurosis, rendering it more creative.

How does this reanimation of creativity take place? Via the reanimation of the power of the spoken word and listening. Is the psychoanalyst in some way a magus of listening? The psychoanalytical cure and in some cases psychotherapy produce within the subject a reanimation of the creative capacities at work within speech and listening. Does the spoken word have this power - a magical one - of healing, killing, building or destroying? Some words reanimate, others immobilize, or kill. Does psychoanalysis not lead us to observe what are magical, or supernatural, conversions? The Persian Magi, religious men, poets, philosophers, interrogated the stars and dreams. The magi are interpreters who make use of various techniques. Poetry creates and deconstructs images within the hollowing-out of words.

The power of the spoken word that knows not, is unaware, of what it says

Interpretation becomes possible on listening to speech that is unaware of what it says. Association is saying whatever goes through one's mind. In order to associate, one must accept the idea of letting go of all logical reasoning. If this model is necessary and beneficial in the treatment of neurotics, it can be dangerous in the treatment of borderline patients. Psychoanalysis, then, is a slow magic, according to Patrick Lacoste (1992: p.118): "… it's a sort of magic that transforms the neurotic fortress into a castle of air. And no, it is not magic, because it takes too much time. It is a slow, or gradual, magic." For the spoken word to regain its meaning and power, speech needs to experience the silence of listening that deconstructs it, that thwarts it even as it accepts or welcomes it.

The floating form of words and the way in which they are heard

In therapy, the spoken word often becomes the object of a game of hide-and-seek with itself: seemingly hidden, or overexposed, within the internal logic of a sentence, an unexpected meaning can make itself heard via a turn of phrase, as if borne out by the listening capacity of the person opposite. Within this curious experience, the spoken word may suddenly reveal or rediscover its own poetic reserve, its very metaphorical strength. The subject may even surprise himself by de-signifying various functional or everyday markers. The realm of dreams, too long assigned only to the field of nocturnal sleep re-appropriates this language – as if insensitive to its own echo – and teaches us to hear it otherwise, through the reflection of a silent listening that proposes to the ear the effect of a mirror. The subject, who, submerged in his own suffering no longer hears himself, and is even more deaf to the words of others, is able to re-appropriate the sense of play within his own words. A distancing of meaning, a distancing of experience, a distancing in time… Such is the curious anachronistic temporality of the therapeutic arena! What age might one have in the spoken word of dreams ? Here, the experience of the creativity of both language and memory takes place within a process that inherently implies the presence of the other. It allows a direct and immediate exchange of both meaning and feelings or affect. This exchange is known as transfer.

If artistic creativity offers the artist a potential space that allows the projection, both within and via the work, of feelings and symbols that cannot be represented otherwise, the work itself is only delivered up to the eye of others once complete. Through this undertaking of the physical creative act, the Ego gives form to a specific object whose statute is never entirely external. Within this solitary endeavour the system of para-excitement is one that needs to be solid in order that the ego not be submerged by the work itself. Here there is no other, if not the foreign object under creation. If certain works may permit an off-loading, or even the sharing of the affective life, they do not have the same specific intensity as the spoken word addressed to a designated listening protagonist. The role of creativity, in art and in therapy, is inherently different. While a work of art may be vehicle to a veritable self-therapeutic power, (art-)therapy remains a hetero-therapeutic undertaking. In order for the necessary healing to be possible, it requires two protagonists. And it would be naive to believe that it is only the therapist who heals the patient! It is a human experience of sharing where each learns from the other, through the other. And yet it is the patient who pays the analyst! When the therapist is not on form it is often his patients who support him. The word *patient* is interesting as such, for it is often the *patient* who teaches the therapist *patience*, that is to say the art of time. In this exchange it is often he who thinks he is giving who in fact receives. What does the therapist then bring if not the vagueness of his listening, a memory impregnated by a particular culture, where the very scarcity or reserve of his words lends them a greater strength?

In French, ausculter, (to sound), and écouter (to listen) have the same Latin root (auscultare). To *sound* (the medical term in English is auscultation), is diagnostically to listen to the sounds of the body (using the ear or a stethoscope) – breaths, wheezes – in the chest, the heart, the veins or arteries, as an indication of their condition. 'Sounding' allows the doctor to access or pick up on sounds (of the organs) that had previously remained hidden. The dictionary Littré notes that to *sound*, in this sense, also signifies *to have faith*, *to listen surreptitiously*, and finally, more surprising, *to obey*. Thus the way one listens to a *sounding* is attentive, endows faith in the power of the word, is transgressive and capable of obedience. From this basis, may we advance the idea that the psychoanalyst is s/he who, rather than sounding the patient's body, sounds the body of words that is the patient's speech? How can one interpret a dream if one is incapable of hearing the body of words of a dream? When the flesh of the dream is inscribed in speech, the images that built up are invited to vaccilate, to explode, to burst apart, to remind humanity that where an image seems certain, in truth blindness strikes. In the same way, in English, *to listen* from the old English hlysnan, evokes the notion of hearing, of paying attention, but also of obedience. If there is not actual regression via listening, can one speak of a vagueness, a floating form of listening? Without the aptitude to regress within listening, to hear the mythological sounds of Eros and Thanatos, there is no analyst, only a usurper with the pretensions of his own Ego.

Wandering within listening, is to break with the very spirit of the sentence, break away from narrativity, or from any temporal continuity. One must learn to listen to the very sound as closely as possible, to the breach of the self. For it is the words within speech, more than any blinding images, that give the tone of these noises, shadows and reflections of the soul – generators of a certain contact. Regressing within listening implies a resonance from within: the whole body becomes a chord, a taut skin, membrane, or instrument. To hear sound, is to offer oneself as an open structure, living from within, like an acoustic space capable of reflecting images. Listening to language is not a chance undertaking! No doubt, one must know how to implicate oneself within the act of listening in the sense that forgetting reaps an awaiting. It is not a distracted or dispersed listening, but on the contrary a concentrated listening, very precise, like an acute attentiveness to what might come forth, what can be accepted or greeted. For Nancy, listening convokes a profound disposition that matches the depth of the resonating drum, which is no other than the body in its entirety: "To be attentive, is to be always at the edge of meaning or within the meaning of a limit and an extremity" (Nancy 2002: p. 21). This disposition of listening invites psychological activity both to forget time in order to become memory, to distance appearance in order to approach the very spirit, and to deconstruct form the better to interpret what is unformed. Of course, in the case of borderline patients, this listening becomes on the contrary an integrative listening.

Taking the time to listen

Leaving words the time to wander, to constitute their own space-time. A form of listening that doesn't rush or hurry in an effort for memorization is essential in the psychotherapeutic process : for by trying too willfully to uncover what is hidden, one risks the conscious ordeal of the trauma of amnesia, which nonetheless preserves the survival of memories. In the film Fellini's *Roma*, from the very moment when we discover the wonderful frescoes that had previously remained walled-up, everything is covered over by a white dust. There is that moment when, after the extraordinary discovery (frescos, bas-reliefs, statues, mosaïcs in a Roman house from two thousand years ago), the conservation that had been made possible through burial, no longer protects. If this psychological material has remained alive, preserved by resistance and amnesia, the posture recommended by Fédida in the psychological treatment of depressed patients, would rather be that of a trans-passible listening, allowing what comes forth through speech the right to appear in its own time. The risks of a forced searching are no doubt not unlike what he calls the "melancholy memory" whose particular violence resides in the fact that " deprived of the living perception of time - it stifles and buries what it tries to reanimate. Obsessive memorisation could be the expression of agony" (Fedida 2000: p92). The clinical sequence described by Fédida (*Les bienfaits de la dépression*) with the patient John is enlightening: "But here, he would learn the presence of someone who asks nothing of him" (p.104). The patient can then express at his own rhythm, no doubt in the way in which he tries to build himself a rhythm and internalize the sensation of time, time that will allow the creation of a space, a gap permitting a play, a movement. Unlike the vision that touches the object, listening favors the interval between the object and its representation.

Voice, presence, breathing, atmospheric elements

"I'd recognize him anywhere!" The expression is a banal one; in the recognition of a face it accords primacy to the image. By what elements do we recognize a familiar person ? The observation of very young children shows that babies take their bearings very early according to the sensorial qualities of the voice. In *The Odyssey*, after so many years of separation, the dog Argos recognizes Ulysses, his master, no doubt by sense of smell; his old nurse Eurykleia by his thigh-wound; Penelope, finally, by the secrets of the marriage bed. We clearly see by this example how recognition operates on the basis of multiple clues; smell, scars, sex... proofs of the flesh. Here again, the visual function doesn't seem to be primordial. The son Telemachus recognizes his father (despite having seen him little) by his *voice saying his name*. Perinatal psychopathology shows that in cases where a mother lacks a capacity for the self-perception of her child's vocality, this doesn't allow the child to recognize his own voice in the voice of the mother. Didier Anzieu (2007) developed these questions remarkably in his article on *The Sonorous Envelope of the Self*. He reminds us of the precedence of the sonorous mirror over the visual mirror as present in the myth of Narcissus. As Echo dries up and perishes, leaving nothing to be heard but a plaintive voice repeating the final syllables, Narcissus is consumed in the mirror of his image. The sonorous space is the first psychological space. By noting some of the pathogenic effects of the sonorous mirror, Anzieu invites psychotherapists to take into consideration certain sonorous qualities of the voice. He reminds us how frequently the voice of the mother of a schizophrenic produces a sensation of unease in the doctor or therapist: "... a voice that is monotone (ill-rhythmed), metallic (without melody), harsh (with a predominance of the low register, creating, in the listener, a confusion of sounds and the sentiment of being intruded on)" [p.84]. He invites us notably to pick up on certain qualities:

> Discordance Brusqueness: at times insufficient, at times excessive, going from one extreme to the other in a way that is both arbitrary and incomprehensible Impersonalness: it is a voice that gives no information about the feelings of the speaker. When the person speaks, one might be hearing the voice of a machine into which the programme of certain telephone operators – a little like a hotline – has been introduced.

Hearing the texture of a voice, the timbre, the tonality (minor, major) the colours (sparkling, dull, lacklustre), the breath, the respiration, the rhythm, the movement animating the word, is in a certain way to *hear the music* within the words. We might advance the hypothesis according to which a culture of musical listening favours an openness to this way of listening in psychotherapy. And yet... Freud hated music, while certain music-lovers would hear nothing of a psychoanalytical listening! But for those analysts who are musicians, it is probable that they find in musical listening an alternative resource to fall back on when the simple use of logos seems insufficient for something of a human contact to be maintained with the patient. Hearing and receiving these forgotten voices, according them both attention and patience. The tone of words is essential when we want to hear what goes unsaid. Sometimes an "everything's fine", accompanied by an exaggerated smile, falls apart and unravels as soon as one lingers on the tone, the texture and timbre of the voice. These remains, murmurs, sounds that overflow and envelop the communicating word, constitute a surround that gives the tone. Sometimes, within a discourse that is cold, clear, argumented, sure of itself, wanting to occupy the whole space, I hear something of a complaint, of a *whine*, of a minor tonality. Like another music that transpires alongside the pronounced words. One could almost speak of a musical accompaniment. The verbal message is enveloped in a certain manner. Listening in this sense is an experience of breaking away, of a distance that suddenly makes its appearance, and at the same time, an experience of closeness. Listening holds itself close to its place of emergence. The ear, like a window that is open onto the far-off and the invisible, is invited to open up to what is outside in order to resonate within.

Interpretation: Favouring the interval, the gap without which there is no interpreter

An interpreter: from the Latin interpres – etis, an intermediary, broker, chargé d'affaire then commentator, oral translator. The interpreter is he who makes understood that which remained hidden. Etymology indicates that to interpret comes from Inter and the extinct verb *Pres* signifying to buy or to sell which would have been related to the word pretium (price). *Giving a price to what is in-between, is to give a value to the interval that allows the movements of Eros.* The symptom requires being considered as in-between two entities, or bodies (that in-between where Joyce perceived the coming forth and disappearance of writing). Fédida, like Nancy, underlines the passive-active power of listening: the capacity for welcoming, receiving, taking form, a very active role in Aristotle's theories on power. Listening in the sense of being receptive to a form, to the modification of appearance. The therapist, via the regression of listening, learns little by little to change form by being receptive to what is unformed within speech.

In this bursting forth of presence, in these apparitions, at the same time a disappearance is also at play. If I stay with my Ego as a therapist, I can hear nothing. In order to reach this stage of creation à deux, one yet needs to be able to regress. If my will for understanding is too strong, I lose the capacity to hear something of madness. *Everything takes place as if it were necessary to retain forgetfulness in order to render these apparitions possible, for if it is not possible to capture forgetfulness, it is impossible to retain forgetfulness.*

Interpretation is to go in the direction of an interval: a stretched interval; and it is precisely when it aims for a form as distant as possible that it may touch on the intimate. Restoring its dream-like dimension to speech is to allow the most foreign of forms (the least logical, the least willful, the least familiar, the most informed of known dialects) to touch upon the very intimacy of psychological life.

References

Anzieu, D. (2007) L'Enveloppe Sonore du Soi. In : Catherine Chabert (ed.) *Psychanalyse des Limites,* Paris, Dunod, pp. 67-89.

Estellon, V. (2007) Ecouter, Interpréter avec Pierre Fédida. In : Jacques André (ed.) *Humain/ Déshumain, La parole de l'œuvre.* Paris, PUF.

Fédida, P. (2000) *Par où commence le corps humain.* Paris, PUF

Fédida, P. (2001) *Les bienfaits de la dépression.* Paris, Odile Jacob

Lacoste, P. (1992) *Contraintes de pensée, contraintes à penser. La magie lente.* Paris, P.U.F., coll. Psychopathologie, 1992, p.118.

Nancy, J.-L. (2000) In : Peter Szendy (ed.) *L'Ecoute.* Paris, L'harmattan, IRCAM, Centre Pompidou) p. 314.

Nancy, J.-L. (2001) *L'il y a du Rapport Sexuel* , Paris, Gallilée.

The Creative Arts Therapies: Playing in the Space Between

David Read Johnson

I hear the sound of the clock, the repeating sound, *tick*, and then the second sound, the second sound, *tick*, it is the same sound, it is the same sound, but no, now I sense a difference, there is a difference between the sounds, tick, and tick. What is this difference? The second tick is *later* than the first tick, the difference is *time*... time arises from the perception of difference between the ticks. I hear the ticks, I do not hear time, where is time?

I am walking and I place my foot on the ground, this is a step, and then I place my other foot on the ground, another step. What is this difference between the two steps? The second one is *further* than the first: another difference erupts in my mind: *space*. Space is the difference between the two steps. Where is space?

There are two things I see. There is a difference between them. What is the difference? Shape! I name one shape a triangle. I name the other shape a circle. Where is shape?

I see two people. There is a difference between them. I call one a mother. I call the other a child. How do they differ? They differ in their role, in identity.

Time and space and shape and color and role arise out of the perception of difference: they are unseen and lay between the ticks and shapes and roles.

Preference

Now as soon as difference is noted, *preference* follows. This is what the Buddha said. For if there is difference, then the whole has been split and each sound and color and shape and person is incomplete. And this incompleteness arises within us as *desire*. We prefer the blue to the red, the mother to the child, or the Caucasian over the Asian. And this urge that arises informs our next action: in art, in deciding the next stroke of the paintbrush, in music the next note that must be played, in drama the next gesture; for as soon as difference is perceived and preference is evoked, that is when we hear the next note or see the next color or shape, *before* we play it or paint it or act it. This is how the tick becomes tock, and why the pessimist hears *tick, tock*, while the optimist hears *tock, tick*.

Territory

And it follows from desire that we wish to bring the preferred closer to us and leave the unpreferred further away, and in this division *territories* are created, through near and far, and the major territories that arise are our body, our mind, our self, the Other, and in space: here and there, and in time, the past, and present and future. All our roles are territories, organized into larger role repertoires, these large tectonic plates that move slowly up, across, and back into being, providing us with the illusion of stability.

The most enduring territory is our body: each day I awake into it again, and see these teeth, these eyes, this hair, and remember this history, again, as I walk into rooms I need not speak or introduce myself for I am recognized, oh that sometimes I could escape this particularity and become mist, fog, a fly on the wall, an eye in the sky, to cloak myself in another's form, an invisible man! But this has yet to happen to me as much as I may have longed for this, it is because I am body that my impulse to move my arm must soon come to a halt, for my arm can only go so far, (though in my mind the movement continues on), to keep it moving I must first return it to my trunk and then set out again, only to be reined in again, and again, repetition, shore, bank.

History

The transformation of these territories over time becomes *history*. These territorializations of desire collect and are stabilized and defended over time, through history, as well as disrupted, invaded, and transformed. They become what we know of as *reality*; these are the grand narratives that appear to define the world we know; this is how reality is constructed out of difference.

Border Regions

But there are other types of territory that lie at the edges, for territories are not only defined by their capitals, but also by their border regions, frontiers, dark forests and misty marshes, where uncertain encounters with the Other may occur.

I know that we all look up at the sky and God knows what anyone sees when they look up there, especially at night, but what my father most often saw was Draco the Dragon, which he carefully pointed out to me on many a night in my youth. Its head of three stars begins near the Big

Dipper and then a series of stars wrapping around the Big Dipper between it and the Little Dipper and then, on certain nights, ending in a tail near the horizon. Now I will make a wild speculation that no one who had not been told previously about Draco the Dragon would be able to see it. In fact, of the eighty some established constellations in the sky, perhaps only three or four might be identified by an uninitiated seer. For the most part, truth be told, there are only a bunch of randomly separated stars up there, in no particular order, and there is certainly not a Dragon there. I mean if I looked up and saw a moving, living fire-breathing Dragon in the sky, that would have been different!

But there is not. Draco the Dragon the constellation certainly exists, but where? Not There, in the sky, but Elsewhere. Draco the Dragon is an idea or image that serves as the center or ground or root or basis or identity of those few points of light, it is this that each of these points share with each other and no other stars.

In contrast, another object in the sky often seen is the Full Moon, an object that my father abhorred because it obscured Draco the Dragon, but nevertheless is probably more widely appreciated. Unlike Draco, 100% of an uninitiated public viewing the sky would identify the Moon as an object, and if I ask them, "Where is the Moon?" all would declare that the Moon is There, not elsewhere. My father would be very distressed to hear that the Moon is There and Draco is Elsewhere.

My answer to this dilemma is simply that Draco must be elsewhere because he is not *all* there, that is, he is suggested by only a few points along his sinuous body and thus it is his *absence* that gives rise to a center elsewhere. Not only that, but to maintain my view of Draco I need to constantly suppress my perception of the many other points of light that surround him but that don't fit in well with Draco, so my seeing Draco involves seeing things that are not there and not seeing things that are there, a most exhausting and dubious task.

Thus Draco is only a symbol, and the symbol exists at the boundary between the seen and unseen, the present and the absent, the given and the possible, and it is the difference between the symbolic and the real that gives rise to the transcendant, called the imagination, heaven, illud tempus, liminal space, or the playspace. Thus it is the simultaneous presentation of the real and the unreal which gives us the imaginative world, and the creative arts.

Instability

Unfortunately all territories, or as the Buddha said, combinations, are turbulent and impermanent. They are unstable because despite all our best efforts to stabilize our concepts of reality and identity, the rapid and constant fluctuations of difference and desire serve to disturb and mix them, especially at their boundaries and edges. Yes the natural world consists of flux and mixture; it is we who attempt to stem the tides of change and bring order and territory into existence.

Let us consider a map of the world, a well-known image to us. All the countries are represented. Their boundaries are clearly demarcated. But in what way do these boundaries exist? Now imagine a photograph of the world as viewed from space. No longer do we see clearcut divisions; no longer are the countries marked in uniform colors; this world appears to have great variation! If we view another photo from space of a populated area, we would see how the farmlands and city blocks have been neatly divided and clearly bordered; this is called private property! It seems Man and God divide things differently.

God made the first territories when he divided the darkness from light. But how did he do this? Like this?

Or this?

Certainly the first way of doing this is less ambiguous! In the second, where do we draw the line? When does Day become Night? Where does Europe become Asia? The Great Walls and Iron Curtains and Security Fences in China, Korea, Europe, Israel, and Texas are placed on top of a continuous flow of land and culture that in the end will outlast them.

What kind of relations do I have with others around me? Like Figure A? Or Figure B? When does Mine become Ours become Yours? Good fences make good neighbors yes, but not particularly good lovers. Intimate human relationships are characterized not by linear boundaries and secure borders, but by continuities and mixtures and flow at the edges. Their boundaries are more variegated and dimensional.

And indeed, the creative arts arise from the ambiguous playground of the transitional space, where self and other are simultaneously present, not regions of clarity and structure.

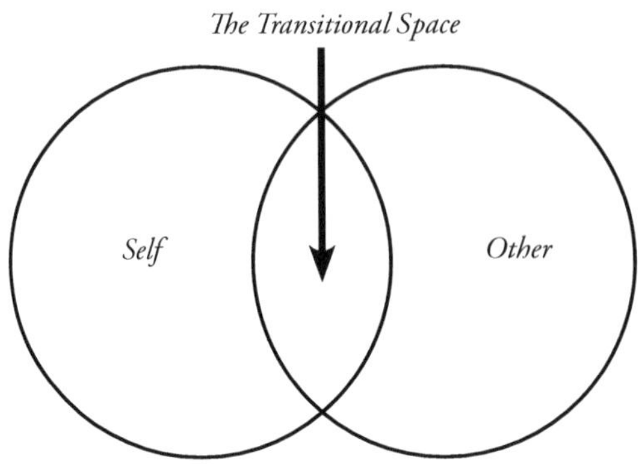

In this interpersonal environment where the child's thought and action mix with the parent's, the beginnings of what will become the capacity for empathy, intimacy, creativity, magic, play, and indeed imagination itself are formed, where capacities for mobility, reversibility, and flexibility are forged, serving as the foundations of what we now call resilience.

These capacities will form of course, if unimpeded by the impact of psychological trauma, which betrays the child's innocent trust in the intermediate area between self and other; the child now pulling back from Us and You, leaving them with only Me.

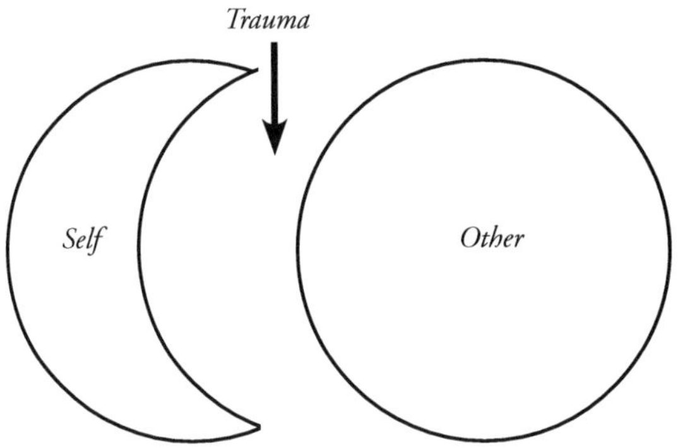

Here is where the heavy border is constructed with its fearful guards and easily triggered alarms. Here is where the sense of absence, the bottomless hole, the unquenched thirst, and the constant quivering arise.

Having been forced to accommodate to the desires of the perpetrator, the child reacts against every new demand to accommodate, whether at school or work or from loved ones, crippling their adaptation to the world. Any new state that proposes an overlap with another's inner territories is avoided, the child now rejecting claims of empathy, pushing aside the benefits of intimacy.

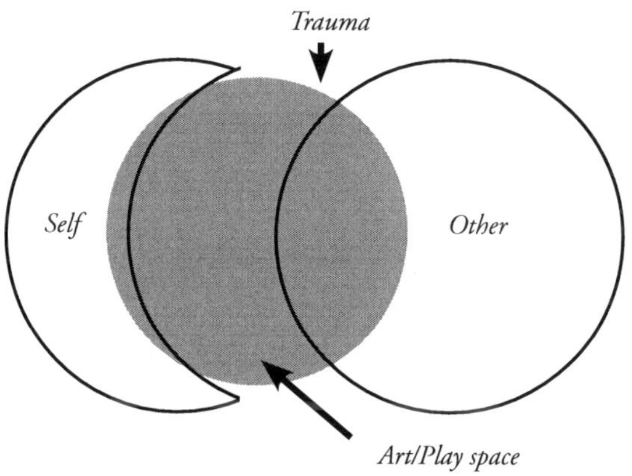

Treatment will need to lower the child's fear of their traumatic memories, by pointing out the discrepancy between the past and present, and to help them accept new demands for accommodation that will not harm them, by introducing them to situations in which self and other, reality and imagination interpenetrate.

Trauma is forced accommodation resulting in:

- Rigid interpersonal boundaries
- Ressistance to further accommodation
- Demands for others to accommodate
- Avoidance of mixed or overlapping states
- Impairment in ability to differentiate among variations of stimuli

Though many forms of treatment accomplish these tasks, the creative arts therapies are especially ripe arenas for this work to take place, for the arts use symbols which, like Draco the Dragon, lie across the boundary of inner and outer, the seen and unseen. The arts provide that canvas or stage necessary for the repair of the broken connection experienced by trauma survivors, where the first tentative steps towards taking down the Wall can occur. They are a bridge that allows the imaginal and liminal worlds to reveal themselves. *The arts make the absent present, whereas trauma makes the present absent.* Trauma in fact may be viewed as the antithesis to art: trauma sucks the present into the unseen, the trauma schemas enveloping larger and larger portions of the person's life. Characters on the stage and images on the canvas are *larger than life* while trauma victims feel reduced, that some essential part of them has been removed or stolen. While the arts take us to the point of catharsis of emotion, trauma leads us to emotional numbing and the cold stare into elsewhere. The arts develop, they move us; trauma repeats, it freezes us; with the arts, we overflow; with trauma, we are hollowed out.

Treatment:

- Lower their fear of their traumatic memories
- Point out the discrepancy between the past and the present
- Help them accept new demands for accommodation that will not harm them
- Introduce mixed states of self and other, and reality and imaginations

There are many forces in this world intent on reminding us of our Deep Fear, and encouraging us to build up our Great Walls and Gated Communities and Security Fences in the name of greater Safety. Healing from trauma requires another sentiment, another courage; another attitude toward boundary. Do we really need to teach our clients to construct border stations and to issue visas to those who wish to come close, or do we show them the pleasures of moving unimpeded across former borders of mistrust and misunderstanding? Do we strengthen their underground shelters or invite them to come out again? Do we warn them against the dangers of downhill skiing, driving a car, or riding a bicycle and tell them they do not need to learn how to do these things, or do we gently assure them that "yes, they can do it" and encourage them, even strongly, to try again?

Yes, it is when the walls and defenses are opened up, when risks are taken, *and no harm takes place*, that a true sense of safety is achieved. And this act is achieved with each creation of the arts/playspace.

It is here strangely, that the arts therapies and the cognitive behavioral treatment for trauma overlap. For what CBT labels as faulty cognitions, are these too narrowly defined, one dimensional boundaries of thought and affect: for the rape victim to not trust *all* men, for the motor vehicle accident victim *never* to re-enter an automobile; for the combat veteran to give up any expression of intimacy. The CBT therapies attempt to do the very same thing that the arts therapies do: to open up the borders between the past and the present, and to be safe. This is what is meant by desensitization.

CBT and Arts-based Methods:

- Imaginal Exposure – guided imagery, play
- Cognitive Restructuring – roleplaying, restorying
- Affect Management – relaxation, exercise
- Resilience Enhancement – creativity, flexibility
- Testimony – performance, exhibitions

As it developed, cognitive-behavioral treatment freely borrowed many of its techniques from the arts and body-oriented fields. By incorporating guided imagery into exposure therapy, role-playing into cognitive restructuring, relaxation into affect management, creativity into resilience enhancement, or performance into testimony, cognitive-behavioral therapy finds itself more closely linked with the arts therapies than has been appreciated.

Both the arts therapies and CBT share deep optimism, and encourage trauma clients to take risks again: to risk intimacy, to risk imagination, to risk embodiment, to risk being, despite the history of injury.

For the world is unstable, yes. The world can be dangerous, yes. Can we learn to lower our fears of these instabilities so that we can reassert our presence? Yes. So let the creative arts therapies be a practice that allows participants to lower their fear over the instability of being, and to approach and allow the ebb and flow of difference and desire, rather than mapping out the territories of role and canonizing history further through story. Let the creative arts therapies be a practice that helps people open their boundary regions between their bodies and others bodies, their minds and others minds, and between the past, present and future, resulting in continuity, mixture, diversity, and animation which in turn give rise to intimacy and presence. Oh how challenging this can be!

Being in Proximity to the Other

We are like two banks of an unseen river which flows between us, lines of becoming arising somewhere upstream and flowing downstream. As we close in on one another, the river moves more rapidly, white water, rapids, turbulence increases, rushing as it were between us, and then when we move apart, the water slows, evens out, lays quiet, almost as if not flowing at all. Proximity!

I turn to my side, away from you, you who enter my space and intrude on my peace, you, who lie next to me, whom I have married or loved or met or seen or withdrawn from, *who breathes as you wish,* whom at times I can't bear, the smell of you, the way you move, the way you deny me. I turn to my side and you turn to your side, and we move apart, all the while keeping the other in sight or in mind, and a strange thing happens, for this sideways movement around each other becomes an orbit, a constant escape which never succeeds, an eternal return, yes, as I walk out the door in the morning and return in the evening, as I turn from you in bed to get some space only to find myself, again, in your arms, as we argue then kiss and make-up, slam doors and send cellphone apologies.

When I and the other allow ourselves to remain in close proximity, in embodied encounter, with the rush of time and space moving between us, then all that the Buddha said can be experienced, for all life is turbulent, all life is impermanent, and flows in an endless stream, dependent origination... and it is in this close proximity, this collection of tremoring vibrations, that our souls light up, incandescent, like the coalescence of dust into stars, or like this gathering of people from far and wide, into this one small space.

We are these banks that encase the stream, these repetitions of identity and name and sensibility that define what is, that give us the solidity we have. Yet we cannot resist the water, we place our feet in the river to feel its flow, as each act is repeated, as each entity affirmed, as each boundary is marked, the Other calls forth, and the lines of becoming rush between us, confusing us, enlivening us, causing all things to rise and fall and turnabout, yes, as we approach the Other, the flow of this lifestream increases, from here to there, and in this here to there we surmise an origin and end, a source and a destination, a home and the frontier.

Oh do we not hear the warning!: "Beware of the Other, beware of the rushing stream, stay back from the shore and its dangers! The rapids may become too turbulent, you could be pulled in, and heavens, could drown or be carried away! Enough with proximity! Enough with becoming! Give me some space! You are driving me crazy! LET ME BE!"

If the turbulence that arises when my encounter with the Other becomes too intimate, first, let me withdraw, gain distance from this awful proximity I have stumbled into, move away from the other shore till it recedes in the distance, as stream becomes lake becomes sea. Let me avert my gaze, let me move to the other side of the room, let me speak of other things, let me speak of things, let me raise problems, let me fall silent, let me turn off the light, let me leave, oh, door, taxi, internet, airplane, the sweetness of departure!

Or perhaps I am not able to leave, or do not want to leave, but simply want to dam up this rushing stream! Yes, to STOP IT! Why let it go on! Let my body be still, let me break these relentless arms of the clock to let time stand still, so yes I will let you hold me, kiss me, know me, only my hand or my face or my mind will go numb, limp, dead, *for You*, because any movement on my part will reveal my choice, my endlessly repeating choice, which is my freedom which is difference which is the stream. So I cannot allow this to begin. No, let me remain frozen in your sweet embrace, and tell you, each time, of my sorrow.

Or perhaps a third urge arises, not to depart from or stop the stream, but to cross over to the other shore! To overcome this river that suddenly becomes an obstacle to me, which means to deny the river, in order to TOUCH or rather to HAVE, the Other. And so a transaction occurs between us, with grasping and clinging and other forms of possession, with hitting and killing and other forms of aggression and violence, with stimulating and rubbing and other forms of sexual contact, with dominating and controlling and other forms of oppression and submission, with performing and exhibiting and pleasing and cajoling, and with saving, caring and hugging and other forms of nurturing, all these things which we do to and with each other.

All these crossings, or transactions, between the banks of the river, between myself and the proximal other, which are the actions of our everyday lives, are not intended to intensify the stream but rather to triumph over it, to bridge it, to nullify it, to deny it, to diminish it. Sex and aggression are instincts, yes, but really they are not desires, for desire is of the river. No, sexual and aggressive acts are the intolerance of desire, they are the wish to end desire, to reach the other shore and to land; they are bridges and landings and invasions of the Other.

And so it may seem that relationships are a hopeless challenge. But that is not true! That the world is unstable and filled with risks not only frightens us, it entices us, for we are drawn to these waterfalls and roller coasters and sky divers and tightrope walkers and surprise parties and haunted houses and water parks and bicycles and, most unstable of all, people! We seek out the edge, we throw our children in the air, we go down to the shore. And ironically, we do what every child does when they arrive at the riverbank or ocean shore... we reach down, grab a piece of the shore, a rock, a stick... and throw it into the water, to watch it sink or float down the river and then we throw another one again. At the ocean shore we build our castle down by the water, always on the incoming tide, so that our failure is assured, where we fight for its survival with all our might until the moment arrives when all hope is lost and the waves crash over our inner walls, and at that moment of impending devastation... we switch sides and with great delight jump up and down on our own castle, joining with the ocean as it takes our treasured home! This is our playspace, where we live through our fears and experience the awe and humility of being here... the playspace lies at the edge of the water as shore or self sinks down into the stream... transitional space. Real space lies away from the water, for protection. We build our real homes away from the risk of flooding, our real world is to be preserved, held onto, as we hold onto our possessions, our children, our spouses, our savings, our careers, ourselves. In contrast we build sandcastles near the water's edge, on the incoming tide, in order to fight for survival, and in order to lose that fight as sea claims our precious possessions. And so in a similar way, we allow our playspace to claim the precious accomplishments of the Self: our roles and stories... in the work we do we take these pieces of ourselves and throw them into the space between us and the client, over and over again, and let them float away, only to look down and find another story, even shinier or smoother than the previous one, and throw it out, hoping perhaps to delay its demise by skipping it once or twice or many times more.

This is what the creative arts therapies can be: throwing sticks in the river, building castles at the edge of the incoming tide, throwing our roles and stories out toward the Other, and having everything carried away.

Conclusion

So our work appears to be about difference and proximity: we engage our bodies in an encounter with our clients, we engage in repetitions of bodies and images and personas and movements and ideas, and we progressively move closer into proximal space while at the same time trying not to freeze, flee, or deny this uprising stream of difference, of turbulence, of feeling, of life that rises between us. Indeed, these are the ways that the client exits the playspace, for at times they need to hold onto something and they do not yet know that they can hold onto us; and when this occurs, we must back away temporarily, and then make our approach again.

We seek an embodied encounter with the Other in which there is equanimity about the turbulence and impermanence of experience in proximity to one another. We seek to make our boundaries more permeable, knowing that elements of the unpreferred will arrive, and accepting that this is the price of intimacy, and of presence.

In the end therapeutic transformation comes down to this: to play with difference and proximity until we feel the illusion of solid ground become the sway of open sea, and learn to delight in it, and fear it less.....but then to go home and wash off our feet, sit down for dinner, tidy our rooms, and go to bed after saying our prayers, and wait for the next day and the next repetition, for each departure becomes a return; the hand that tucked me into bed lives in my hand, as I put my son to sleep, again and again, and the sun sets, and then rises again, just as I move away, and come back to you, day after day, being like the earth's eternal attempt to free itself from the sun, foiled again.

In the space between the ticking sounds and beating hearts, time and space, you and I arise, and all the rest seems to follow on from there.

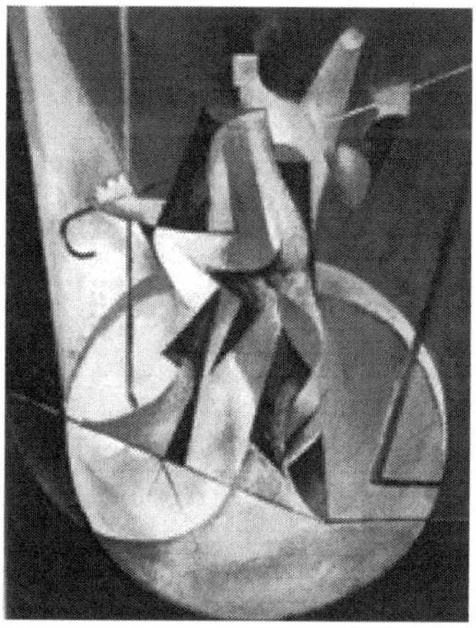

The Arts Therapies: The Problem for the Potential for Change when there is No Space Between

La question du « potentiel de changement » lorsqu'il n'y a pas d' « espace intermédiaire »

Edith Lecourt

Synopsis

The author develops reflections on the themes *the space between* and *the potential for change*, and comments on their place and function in the practice of the arts therapies in connection with authors such as Winnicott, Bion, Meltzer, Bick, Bollas and Anzieu. The *potential for change* is a fundamental hypothesis, or more, a basic assumption for all arts therapists. This basic assumption is that there exists in each client a potential for change, even if nothing in the attitude, the behavior and even the client's history, seems to relate to such a possibility. This is not a scientific position. To have some efficacy it must be like a necessary belief. It is the motor of our work. We should recognize that very often it is linked to an all-powerful personal fantasy: feeling able to work a miracle! This link has to be analyzed during training. But the basic assumption stays as essential. It is a basic condition for developing *the space between. The space between* is a fundamental condition of the therapeutic setting itself in the process of the development of *the potential for change*. In many pathological situations we will have first to create the conditions of *a space between* inside the art therapeutic relationship.

Résumé:

L'auteur développe sa réflexion sur les notions d' « espace entre » (espace intermédiaire) et de « potentiel de changement », et commente leurs places et fonctions dans la pratique des arts thérapies , en relation avec des auteurs tels que Winnicott, Bion, Meltzer, Bick, Bollas et Anzieu. Le « potentiel de changement » est pour tous les arts thérapeutes une hypothèse fondamentale, ou, plus encore, un principe de base. Ce dernier est qu'il existe chez chaque client un potentiel de changement, même si rien dans l'attitude, le comportement et l'histoire même du client ne semble en relation avec une telle possibilité. Ceci n'est pas une position scientifique. Pour avoir une certaine efficacité cela doit se présenter comme une croyance nécessaire. C'est le moteur de notre travail. Nous devrions reconnaître que, très souvent, ceci est en lien avec une fantaisie personnelle de toute puissance : se sentir capable de faire un miracle ! Ce lien doit être analysé au cours de la formation. Mais le principe de base reste essentiel. C'est la condition pour le développement de l' « espace intermédiaire ». Cet espace est une condition fondamentale du dispositif thérapeutique lui-même dans le processus de développement du « potentiel de changement ». Dans beaucoup de situations pathologiques nous avons tout d'abord à créer les conditions d'un « espace intermédiaire » à l'intérieur de la relation art thérapeutique.

Key words:
Arts therapies, music therapy, therapeutic change, transitional space, transformational object

INTRODUCTION

The space between and the potential for change sound like familiar and common sense propositions in arts therapy circles. Because it seems evident that in the arts therapies there is a space between and there is a potential for change. We will question this assumption. As most of the papers on these subjects base this assumption upon a range of different evidence, I shall be explaining why, for me, from my clinical experience, there is no such evidence. I also wonder if the fact that these two propositions have been placed side-by-side means that the space between is a potential for change? I could fully agree with this positive perspective. But the fact is that, working with our clients, we often observe that there is no space between and sometimes also we are also in doubt of a potential for change. I will develop these ideas through three propositions:

I - FIRST PROPOSITION: THE POTENTIAL FOR CHANGE IS A BASIC ASSUMPTION FOR ALL ARTS THERAPISTS

The proposition of a *potential for change* can be considered through four topics: art itself, the client, the setting, and the arts therapist.

Art as a potential for change

This is the main idea supported by most of the relevant papers. I will only choose one theoretical reference: Bollas' ideas on change. Christopher Bollas is a British psychoanalyst. He wrote about what he called *the transformational object*, which I find especially inspiring for the arts therapists (Bollas 1989). Bollas has shown that the first relational development is also the moment the baby experiences the first and most massive changes, physical and psychic changes together (without being able to distinguish them), changes that occur through the first daily experiences of being cared for. During these experiences the newborn finds himself successively: turned upside down, turned round, sometimes thrown up, or sitting on the mother's lap, lying on one side, on the other, standing face to face, lying on the back (discovering the ceiling), on the belly etc. Each of these spontaneous movements of necessary caring produces huge transformations of the baby's internal and external worlds. The baby discovers a new world outside and new sensations inside. This observation sounds like a complement of Winnicott's concepts of handling and holding (Winnicott 1971).

All of these corporal transformations and the emotions associated create each time new perceptive worlds. For this author this experience of transformations is the origin of our representation and our demand for change, in terms of a magic, massive and passive change; the origin of our huge expectation towards therapy. And we expect that the therapist, like the mother, does the work! I will add, for our reflection, that this experience is, for the baby, the first space organizer.

To develop and refine his idea, Bollas proposes to qualify the mother, in this case, as *a transformational object*, as she is the agent of the transformation (Bollas 1989). And if I choose to present these ideas of Bollas here, it is because it is the author's sense of the experience of change experienced through the perception of an artistic work. In each case it is a global change, a massive impression. For instance, I have this experience when I visit an exhibition of paintings, when I encounter an opera that makes me feel a change of my mental and physical states. Sometimes also, at the end of my visit, on my way home, I observe that my perception of the world around me has changed. In other situations, for example, I listen to a piece of music and suddenly observe that my mood is changing massively, feeling melancholy or joy.

This reflection can be completed by Meltzer's publication on aesthetics (Meltzer & Harris Williams 1988). I don't agree with the idealization of the mother's internal world (I am not sure of such an interpretation), but we have to think of the quality of these very first massive changes and the way some of them will become an artistic feeling.

So the conclusion could be that artistic pieces have the potential to create changes that resonate with the very first changes we have experienced as a baby.

Let's now look at the second point:

The client's potential for change: observation, assumption, or belief

If the assumption of the existence of a potential for change sounds like an idea easy to grasp when we work with young children, it is much more difficult with some adults and with elderly clients. Because of their age and their state of development it seems we might assume, for young clients, that there is a potential for development, for change. And this could still be the case even if the sessions of art therapy have no efficacy at all!

But this assumption can conflict with objective data for some of our clients as, for example, with clients suffering from Alzheimer's dementia. And, in these cases, we need more than an assumption (which has to be demonstrated), we need a belief, the belief in a potential for change whatever the client's situation is (a belief does not need to be demonstrated).

It happens also, sometimes, that we have to work with a client who has received a critical medical prognosis, and we still work with the idea (the belief) of a potential for change! (HIV, cancer, coma etc.) In these cases, the potential for change has not to be objective (there could be no assessment of it), but it needs to exist in the subjective position of the arts therapist.

But there is, however, at least one exception: last work at the bedside of the dying. We have also to respect a position of renouncement or a refusal of change. Change is not a value for itself. In some situations there might be no need for change, but only to be sustained, to be listened to, to be assured companionship.

We have also to consider that the question is not only on the part of the client, but also on the part of the arts therapist.

The potential for change introduced by the setting

The setting of an arts therapy is thought to be, and practically prepared as, a *good environment* (with reference to Winnicott (1971)) for a process of change. We are responsible for these necessary conditions of our work: the physical space, the institutional conditions, the choice of method, of material, etc. Paradoxically, arts therapy sessions cannot be improvised even if improvisation is the method used. The setting of the different arts therapies is a creation of a particular space which offers the potential for change. It is the organization of the space within the therapeutic relationship and of the circumstantial space of the session.

The art therapist's potential for accepting changes

Is the arts therapist open to changes occurring through the sessions? Is he/she prepared to identify and accept these changes? Even if the outcome were to be the end of the sessions, the conversion to verbal therapy, or the transfer of the client to a colleague, etc.? This is uncertain, because arts therapists find their motivation in this especial position of help – which they like – and this motivation (vocation?) could create a resistance to accepting the client's change with its consequences for the art therapist. This concerns also the problematic issue of the end of the arts therapist's work with a client. We all know that the willingness to help can be an obstacle in this professional work, as it is a personal narcissistic position. Personal work and supervision are the tools by which we open and keep the door open for our clients.

Finally I think that there could not be arts therapy without the belief in a potential for change, on the client's side, and the acceptance of changes and their consequences, on the therapist's side.

II - SECOND PROPOSITION: THE SPACE BETWEEN IS PART OF THE POTENTIAL FOR CHANGE

The space between is situated at a level other than that of the potential for change. For the arts therapist it is a question of setting, a technical point about the physical space in the session and within the relationship. It is also the question of the choice of the mediation. The physical space is often a support, a metaphorical figure, of the psychic *space between*, so that it has resonances with psychological development and with the pathology. I will consider now these two points.

The space between and the development of the Ego: a structural component of the psyche

D. W. Winnicott's (1958) work on this question of space - transitional, cultural spaces – is well known: how this space develops itself from the fusion with the mother to the capacity for the child to play in the presence of the mother (Winnicott 1958a). The creation of the transitional object sustains this progression. W. R. Bion (1962) has also developed the idea that the mother thinks and dreams for the baby and on the baby's state, offering her adult psychic space as long as the baby needs it to create his own psychic space.

I shall refer now to Didier Anzieu's (1985) framework. Didier Anzieu is an influential French psychoanalyst who was especially attentive to somatic difficulties and to regressive states. So, as a psychoanalyst, he was confronted not only with an analysis of the psychic contents (as in traditional psychoanalysis with neurotic patients) but also with the question of containment (Bion's concept). He used to offer metaphors to help our representation of psychic processes. Following Esther Bick (1968), he developed the image of the skin, of a *psychic skin* which, like the physical skin, has a protective function, a function of limit, a function of articulation between the interior and the exterior of the psyche, a function of relation and many others etc. This *psychic skin* is more than an analogy with the physical skin, because the link between body and psyche is not analogical but metaphorical. It refers to the intimate experience of the skin, endeavouring to elaborate mentally this experience.

Anzieu (1895) distinguished a structure with two sheets: one sheet in relation with the exterior, the other with the interior. And even if the two sheets are very close, to compose the psychic skin (or the Ego skin) between the two sheets there needs to be a space. He observed that in several pathologies this space doesn't exist or, on the contrary, this space is too large. He analyzed as precisely as possible these forms of pathology. The construction of this space roots in the mother-child relationship, in the way the baby's environment responds to the baby's needs. When these responses are given in a fusional way, responding immediately and sometimes misunderstanding the needs, the baby has no space to build his Ego. On the contrary, when the response is too late, the baby is lost and has to construct himself without the material necessary. We recognize in this last case the pathology of a *false self* as Winnicott (1971) called it. And we observe here that space and time are going together: a deregulation in time is expression of a lack of space.

The Ego skin, with its double sheet, is the indispensable construction to receive and contain psychic material (perceptions, representations, thoughts). In many of the cases that we meet in the arts therapies, these first bases have not been achieved: there is no *space between* to work with. The arts therapist has first to offer a creative condition to help the development of a structured psychic space (cf. the "first space organizer" mentioned earlier).

When there is no space between: an example

Lise is a 50 year old woman suffering for years a psychotic depression. She has been hospitalized twice before her coming to music therapy. As she is a nurse, she is always very well informed about the different therapies. She had read an article on music therapy that made her think that this could be good for her. She is a positive character, she knows what she wants! In this case she asks precisely for receptive music therapy: she wants to listen to music and not to speak (she has a long record of medical interviews)! She cannot even give any useful indication about her musical preferences. She says she needs a full hour of music! She refuses to speak after this listening, to give her impressions. But it happens that she reacts corporally: after one session she belched and commented, "To belch is a sign that it is good"! I was very surprised at this reaction, but she repeated it in other sessions and, after one of them she made a kind of vomiting movement. I observed that each time she had a feeling of frustration (at the silence between two music pieces, or at some empty minutes left at the end of the session, for example) she manifested her displeasure physically.

In this particular case we observe that the demand itself leaves no place, no space for anything else than a fusion in music. The therapist and the pieces of music have no independent existence. Music is absorbed with indifference, like a quantity of milk. In this very regressive state, music was the good or bad milk given by the therapist. Music was also a common envelope (Lecourt 1987) but without the distinction of the two sheets according to Anzieu's analysis. In this situation music couldn't be recognized as a mediator, it was absorbed! There was no such thing as a *space between* either with the music or with the therapist.

After ten sessions (which was my first proposal) she said she felt fully better and that she didn't want/need more!

We consider that her choice of music therapy was linked to her demand of a melting situation (with no space between her and the music pieces, and no space for a relationship – other than fusion – with the arts therapist). This would be more difficult for her with other media such as painting, theatre or even dance, as music has a high potential of fusion.

Lise wanted to feel better with what she had decided and in the way she had decided. She couldn't leave space for something else. Finally she felt better in the way she was ready to. She taught me what listening to music can be for such regressive states. And I also learned, at that time, that simply complying with the patient's demand can result in being limited by the patient's fantasy of being all-powerful.

In summary I conclude that in the arts therapies the absence of the space between can be a consequence of one or several of these following factors: the client's (and sometimes the institution's) pathology, the lack of an appropriate setting, the potential of fusion inherent in the artistic activity, the way the regressive movement is used inside the session, the counter-transference of the arts therapist.

III - THIRD PROPOSITION: THE CLIENT'S LACK OF SPACE BETWEEN IS A THERAPEUTIC INDICATION FOR AN ORIENTATION TO THE ARTS THERAPIES

The arts therapies offer a potential for a *space between*, which can be essential for some clients. But, if the physical presence of a mediator (medium) is the offer of every arts therapist, it says nothing of the reality of a process of mediation, which is something else.

This is a paradoxical situation: there is a trend to fusion in the arts therapies, but the arts therapies offer settings in which a *space between* can be elaborated, opening a potential for change. I will now comment on this proposition.

There is a trend (and a risk) to fusion in the arts therapies:

Fusion is facilitated by a regressive process suggested by our arts therapeutic settings, and especially the non-verbal situation, the group setting (when used) and the artistic mediation itself.

- Our non-verbal mediator (music, painting, dance, drama etc.) has a potential of regressive processes; these regressive processes are generally seen as a possible tool in the therapeutic process (which includes regressive and progressive movements)
- When we use group settings (which was not the case for Lise) we combine two possibilities of regressive processes – non-verbal process and group process – also seen as a tool in the therapeutic process
- Each one of our artistic mediations has a different potential of regressive movement, also linked to the character of the artistic conventions used in the method. For example, free improvisation is more potentially regressive than a structured exercise.

Fusion is not a negative state in the therapeutic process, but fusion has to be part of the process (not a goal), worked through. For the therapeutic objective is not fusion but individuation.

The mediator and the process of mediation

As for Lise there can be a mediator – from an objective point of view - but no process of mediation. It is the work of the arts therapist to create conditions for the development of a process of mediation. In some situations the arts therapist is lacking a *space between* in his/her relationship with the client, and/or in his/her work with the medium. The physical support of a space between, the medium, does not guarantee the process of mediation. The therapist needs special competencies. S/he will find support for that in the arts therapy theory, in the link with professional societies, in supervision, etc. Bion (1962) wrote about the mother's process of thinking the baby's situation. Our theories help us create such a space of thinking inside the session.

Arts therapies are good indications for clients lacking of a *space between*: in this case, the primary aim is to help the client build a space between. But, more precisely, what do we mean by *space between* in painting, dancing, playing music?

In the different settings of the arts therapies, how can we define the *space between*: as a basic condition, as a therapeutic focus, as a therapeutic aim?

I shall try to answer for my specialty: I should say that, in the case of music, the *space between* is a basic condition. I have developed the idea that, from the structural point of view, music is based on the sonorous/musical interval: an interval between two sounds, two notes. In music these two notes are tuned to be at a *good* distance from each other. I use it as a metaphor of the relationship, and I use the musical structure as an elaboration of the structure of communication, in space and time, in simultaneity and continuity. The setting of *sonorous communication* which I have developed is a clinical work on this sonorous process, from unison (fusion) to polyphony in a setting of free improvisation.

The space between is the interval progressively attuned within the relationship. It is very often a therapeutic focus, because it is the condition to discover and develop a potential for change. Using the propositions of Bollas and Winnicott we could write that the process could be to develop the way from the transformational object to the transitional object.

References

Anzieu, D. (1985) *Le Moi Peau.* Paris, Dunod.

Bick, E. (1968) The Experience of the Skin in Early Object Relations. In *International Journal of Psycho-Analysis, Vol 49*

Bion, W.R. (1962) *Aux Sources de l'Expérience.* Paris, PUF.

Bollas, C. (1989) L'Objet Transformationnel. *Revue Française de Psychanalyse vol 4.*

Meltzer, D. and Harris Williams, M. (1988) *The Apprehension of Beauty.* Perthshire:Clunie Press

Winnicott, D.W. (1971) *Jeu et Réalité.* Paris, NRF Gallimard.

Winnicott, D.W. (1958) La Capacité d'être Seul. In : *De la Pédiatrie à la Psychanalyse.* Paris, Payot.

Winnicott, D.W. (1958a) Objets Transitionnels et Phénomènes Transitionnels. In : *De la Pédiatrie à la Psychanalyse.* Paris, Payot.

Lecourt, E (1987) The Musical Envelope. In : Anzieu, D. (ed.) *Psychic Envelopes.* London, Karnac Books.

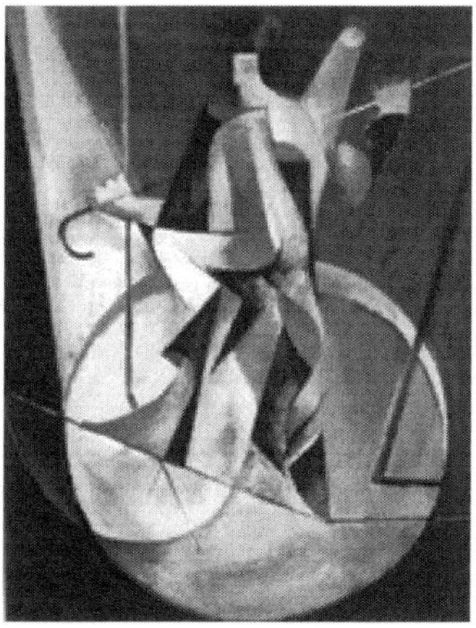

Reflections on Artistic Matter

Marián López Fdz. Cao

Synopsis

This essay explores some ideas around the concept of creation associated with dominance and power over others. Taking this into account, it analyses some fundamental characteristics of modern creation. From there another concept is proposed, linked to caring and sharing, which can subvert the idea of creation and can be a useful space for the dynamics of art therapy.

Sinopsis

El objetivo de este texto es analizar las bases sobre las cuales se consolida en occidente el término creación. A partir de ello el capítulo propone otro modo de comprender ésta, ligada al arte como terapia y la inclusión social.

A partir de la obra de Simone de Beauvoir, *El Segundo Sexo*, ésta autora señala que el origen de la dominación de la mujer y la naturaleza por el hombre parte de una propensión original en la conciencia del ser humano a la dominación del otro, reforzada por el descubrimiento de los instrumentos de metal. Este descubrimiento de los instrumentos del metal supone un "darse cuenta" en la psique de que la naturaleza puede convertirse, de repente en objeto de dominio. La naturaleza, lo Otro, deja de ser el interlocutor, con el cual hay que mediar, comprender y aceptar, a ser el objeto que se modela, domina y responde a nuestras demandas. Si a este descubrimiento se añade que el medio es violento, la fuerza del herrero que somete y da forma a la materia, la metáfora de la creación como violencia contra el mundo está ya construida desde sus albores.

Erigirse como transformador de la materia a través de la fuerza, impone una estructura que será la que se desarrollará a través de los siglos que entiende no sólo la posibilidad de dominar y transformar la naturaleza y lo orgánico, sino de **entender la creación como transformación de la**

materia a través de la violencia.

En la primera parte de este texto se analiza ésta construcción, a partir de diversos autores como Victor Hugo o Gaston Bachelard.

En una segunda parte se propone el pensamiento de Hannah Arendt como inauguradora de otra voz sobre la actividad humana y la creación. A partir de su pensamiento se postula que el proceso creador, unida al pensar poético, puede situarse en la acción arendtiana, frente al concepto de homo faber y trabajo que define. La creación, el proceso creador, se halla cercano a la natalidad, a la pluralidad, y a la imprevisibilidad.

El proceso creador, que deviene en casos producto poético o artístico, no es fabricación pues en el sentido arendtiano, porque ese producto no es estable, durable u objetivo. Sólo la sociedad de cada época puede asignarle esas características, que devienen necesidades de esa sociedad concreta. La persona creadora sabe de la imprevisibilidad, de la fragilidad de su proceso, de la urdimbre desde donde parte, en un magma donde se mezcla el ser y los otros, la individualidad y la pluralidad.

De algún modo, y frente al concepto arraigado en la tradición moderna occidental, existe otra creación que no es dominio, que no está ligada a lo instrumental, a lo utilitario en el sentido más metafórico, que no está ligada al poder sobre los otros. Una creación no dominadora. Una creación con los otros, para sí y los otros, con el mundo, sabiendo del mundo. Una creación que a través de su proceso ininterrumpido y recomenzado una y otra vez ha sabido de su imprevisibilidad y de su irreversibilidad, y ha gozado con ello. Esta es la propuesta de este texto como fundamento del arte y la inclusión y del arte como terapia.

¬

My hope is that this essay will contribute to the understanding of creation from a little-explored point of view or will at least encourage the reader to rethink what we are usually taught about creation at Art School, and how art therapy and social inclusion can be the starting point for inquiry into new concepts and paths in the field of creation.

On revisiting the work of Simone de Beauvoir for other purposes, I discover that in her work *The Second Sex (Le Deuxième Sexe*, 1949*)*, she points out that the origin of man's domination over woman and nature derives from an original propensity rooted in human beings to dominate; a fact which is reinforced by the discovery of bronze instruments/tools.

I should like to add that the discovery of metal instruments implies, in Gestaltic terms, that the male's psyche realises suddenly that he can dominate nature. Nature changes from being a challenging surrounding and environment, to which we must adapt, to an object that can be dominated and adapted according to our will. It is no longer the former, an existence with which we must negotiate and which we must understand and accept if we want to survive. If to this discovery we add an element of violence, like the force of the blacksmith who submits and gives form to matter, the metaphor of creation which is understood as violence against the world can be seen as a quintessential characteristic from the origin of mankind.

Using force to transform matter imposes a structure developed through centuries, which allows not only nature and organic domination, but also understands creation as the result of violent transformation of matter. This foundational fact of the creation concept is widely known as a 'natural' characteristic.

De Beauvoir notes in the third chapter of her work that, before the age of metals, "not having appropriate instruments," man:

> "...feels himself lost among nature and society, passive and threatened, a toy of dark forces. He only dares to conceive himself by identifying himself with the clan: the totem, the manna, the earth are collective realities. The discovery of bronze enables man to discover himself as a creator by doing hard and productive work. As he dominates nature, he is no longer afraid of it and he has the audacity to develop himself as an autonomous being in its uniqueness." (De Beauvoir 1949: p.118)

The forge, the blacksmith's work, allows man to become independent from nature. He can isolate it to master it.

The constitution of the blacksmith - based on Gaston Bachelard's *Earth and the Dreams of Will*

I will now focus on Gaston Bachelard's 1948 work, *La terre et les rêveries de la volonté (The Earth and the Dreams of Will)* quoted by De Beauvoir, as an example of this version of creation.

Matter as a metaphor of resistance

The Earth and the Dreams of Will is part of a vast meditation on earth and imaginings about matter. It talks about hard matter and soft matter, brought together to make a synthesis of forged material that shows, according to Bachelard, a completed work, the work *par excellence* since it uses the four elements. There is, however, a common axis, that Bachelard constantly refers to as "the mastery of the job acquired by working against the matter" (Bachelard 1948: p.17). Bachelard posits that Man – referring to the male gender and not to humankind, as I believe Bachelard has in mind the image of man as a universal concept where woman is not included – is formed and measured according to the matter he works against, and through the strategies he uses to tame it:

> "Resistance is earth's first feature. ... On the threshold of our study, we try to characterize the resistant world." (Bachelard 1948: p.17)

This is why forging, according to Bachelard's interpretation of the male's mind, would embody the most total and complete of occupations:

> "Between the poles of imagining hard and soft materials we have a synthesis of the forged material. There we have the opportunity to show the dynamic values of an entire occupation from the point of view of material imagination, since it uses the four elements of a heroic job that gives man the power of a demiurge." (Bachelard 1948: p.18)

Matter becomes a symbol of hostility to be overcome. It generates in man (sic) the illusion of omnipotence, which in turn helps him to dominate matter:

> "The truth is that the material dreams change the dimension of our forces. They give us the illusion of omnipotence. Those illusions are useful because they encourage us to tackle the matter in depth." (Bachelard 1948: p.34)

Based on the psychology of "against", in the illusion that the "domain against" suggests, Bachelard performs and explains his theory:

> "One of the biggest attractions of the novel of Robinson Crusoe is the story of a working life, an industrious life. In the active solitude, the man wants to excavate the land, drill the stone, carve the wood. He wants to work the matter, to transform it. Man is thus no longer a mere philosopher facing the universe, he is a tireless force going against the universe, against the substance of things." (Bachelard 1948: p.39)

> "Working with the matter, *Homo Faber* is no longer happy setting a geometric mental pattern; he enjoys the inner strength of basic materials and the softness of all the materials that he is to master." (p.42)

At this point, matter is a symbol of resistance; the tool is a symbol of power. Bachelard makes a very interesting excursus on the relevance of tools and their links with aggressive behaviour and anger. He quotes George Blin to synthesize the main elements of psychoanalysing the act of cutting the matter "The virile satisfaction born of the desire to cut should be linked with certain forms of contrite sadism. All integrity provokes us." (Blin cited in Bachelard 1948: p.49)

> "Much of the pleasure of cutting should be reduced here to the pleasure experienced when overcoming an objective resistance: the happiness of being or manipulating the hardest instrument, of performing spontaneously and stamping his style to the raw material that yields. Stunning imperialism of the hardest relief: the plough, the diamond, the dagger and the teeth." (Blin cited in Bachelard 1948: p.53)

The tool, a metaphor of power

The features of a good instrument should be, according to Bachelard, accuracy and strength to fight against the hard material. In this way, we have managed to domesticate animals and other fields of nature. Work and creation is therefore defined and this definition is set from the moment we *fight against* and we start using tools that give us power and control over the resistant material. Bachelard is right when he says image metaphors on this subject largely cover the whole of modern thinking on creation and work:

> "And depending on the matter and its strength and hardness, a sense of skill and power grows in the worker's soul. Skill and power will not be without the other, in the dream side of work, in the illusions of will. The tool requires its union so clearly that if each matter has a coefficient of adversity, every tool determines within the worker's soul a coefficient of domain." (Bachelard 1948:p.63)

No wonder Victor Hugo, in his work *Toilers of the Sea* (*Les travailleurs de la mer, 1866),* compares tools to weapons. In this paper about using power against matter, anger and violence become real, expressed through skills and strength:

> "Work invests in hostility. The noise that annoys excites the worker. He increases the blows of the file, he is aware of the squeaks of matter. Soon he enjoys his power. He laughs at the visitor's nervous looks who covers his ears. ... The cries of matter provoke that liveliness. They are cries of anguish that excite the worker's offensiveness." (Bachelard 1948: p.72)

Not only is creation understood as working against matter, tastes of resistance, domination and power; matter also becomes human: it suffers, it cries... and its cry not only arouses the conscience of the worker-artist, but also makes him 'enjoy' the sight of matter suffering under his tools.

This is a tool that does not destroy, but forges a new tailor-made reality once the matter is tamed under his will:

> "Who has not heard the cries - is it despair or fury? - of tempered steel, the shrill sound of the iron attacked by the deep waters?" (Bachelard 1948: p.163)

In all cases, and from this foundational concept of the principles of creation from its very beginning, there is no dialogue on matter, but domination, sheer desire of power over matter to be overpowered and rendered: the dead mother, and now Bachelard does use a feminine metaphor.

From this point all subsequent interpretations are possible: from the pleasure, pointed out earlier, of knowing that matter suffers under our power, hinting clearly at the need to inflict pain on others against their will, to the unequivocal pleasure of the surrendered matter, lost under the rule of he who knows how to manage it. This metaphor, which still usefully describes human social processes in Western cultures, is often ruthlessly applied to anything considered different, other: nature, impoverished classes, children, women, body...

Asserting a creation concept such as the one described here involves examination of the self, of the world and of things, which have little to do with the dialogue and understanding of matter relationships held by other creation concepts.

My thesis is not necessarily to blame, condemn, or erase other views, deeply rooted in the concept of modern creativity, but to point out that despite this obsessive viewpoint, there are other ways of creating, of interacting with matter.

The creation as opening action – based on Hannah Arendt's concept of action

Hannah Arendt's work *From History to Action (De la historia a la acción, 2008)* states in her chapter "Labour, work and action," (originally published in 1957) the difference between *vita activa* and *vita contemplativa*, pointing out that *vita contemplativa* has always been thought to be of a higher level than action which is considered a means to reaching contemplation.

Additionally, Arendt introduces these two approaches to life, making them dependent on one another and identifying three types of activities related to human beings: *labour*, on which depends all that is needed for man's survival, *work* that generates all things necessary to accommodate the human body and *action* that organises the human life in common, in order to ensure peace, the condition for calm contemplation.

It is remarkable that this chapter's first version was written in 1957 ten years after Bachelard's *Earth and the Dreams of Will* and nine years after De Beauvoir's *Second Sex,* and all after the Second World War. The three of them - each one for its own specific purposes - search for the essence of human activity beyond care-taking, raising and subsistence. More than fifty years later, when the value of care-taking has increased, I believe it is convenient to reconsider Arendt's key concepts from different perspectives, as a new generation thinks about the paradigms of human activity and the creation.

The work

The work of our hands, as something different from our body's physical labour, creates the endless variety of things that add up to become human artifice, according to Arendt. They are not consumer goods, but objects for use, which do not disappear with use. They give the world the appearance of stability that human beings seem to need and in that way seem to provide a certain stability, durability and objectivity. As Arendt says,

> "worldly things are there to stabilize human life, and their objectivity lies in the fact that men, despite their ever-changing nature, recover their identity thanks to their relations with the persistent sameness of objects ... Facing the subjectivity of men stands the objectivity of man-made artifice and not the indifference of nature." (Arendt 1995: p.97)

Therefore, durability and objectivity are featured as elements that transform matter into material:

> "...the material is produced by human hands that have extracted it from its natural place, killing a life... or interrupting a natural process... This element of rape and violence is present during manufacturing, and man as creator of human artifice has always been a destroyer of nature... *Homo Faber* becomes nature's master as he violates and partially destroys part of what was given to him." (Arendt 1995: p.97)

This is how work gives back to man the illusion of control over the world, through a manufacturing process which always has a precise beginning and a specific purpose, unlike labour and action. Man feels like a lord of the world and lord of his actions that are finally predictable, durable and determined. At this point Arendt and Bachelard describe the same process, but from very different points of view. For Arendt, work is not and should not be the highest level of human activity, as it conceals and provokes in human beings illusions of mastery and control beyond the relationship with their fellow beings; reactions which are not needed for the production process. Through work, the final product organizes the entire work process and those involved in it. With work comes the instrumentation of everything else, nature and subject, from the material that justifies violence to nature, to the processes and subjects which become the means to obtain the final product, which in turn becomes a means to create another product, another goal, and so on.

Given this situation, Arendt introduces action as a possible activity linked not to an instrumental one, but associated to ethics and to human solidarity.

The labour

Labour, however, as Arendt states, in its conceptualization is linked to an activity related to the body's biological processes. Through labour, human beings produce the vital things needed to nourish their bodies to keep them alive. And since this vital process is in itself circular, labour's own activity must follow the life cycle and the circular movement of our body functions. This means that labour activity never leads to an end while human life goes on. It repeats to infinity. Therefore we find two features associated with labour: on one hand its dependence on the body and, on the other, its cyclical or repetitive character.

Further, Arendt points us to two more features: firstly, that labour produces consumer goods, and secondly, that to labour and to consume are only two stages of the ever recurring cycle of biological life. This means that labour is linked to the cycle of survival. This is why labour is the less 'durable' of human activities. The products obtained perish in the consumption cycle and return, sooner or later, to the natural process that produced it. Despite being the fruit of human hands, says Arendt, they come and go; they are produced and consumed; they disappear, in harmony with the ever-recurring cyclical natural movement. Hannah Arendt considers these activities "unproductive" and futile, although they generate wealth (Arendt 1995: p.95) and happiness intrinsic to labour.

Consumption, repetition and ending are another three features related to labour.

Arendt gives labour little relevance. It has a certain importance since it satisfies our minimum needs of sustenance, according to the Enlightenment approach and close to a Marxist point of view, but labour cannot be considered beyond these means of sustenance.

Nevertheless, in her texts, Arendt never points out that labour has been one of the elements basically reserved for the female gender and for the impoverished classes. The importance of labour's relevance, related to caring and procreation – and considered as life's own reproduction – and the fact that it has been a female gender task, could have been taken into account by Arendt. To consider how female experience contributes as an 'epistemic privilege' means starting to think from other points of view beyond utilitarian perspectives.

However, there are a number of labour's features (also called "care" in some contexts) I should like to emphasize: it is not durable, it is repetitive, it follows the cycle of life and it has to do with the body. These features seem interesting enough to return to later.

Arendt points out how one of the objectives of the revolution was, according to Marx, "not only the emancipation of the working class, but also the emancipation of human beings from labour", because "the realm of freedom starts only when the realm of labour disappears" and where the immediacy of "physical needs" ends (Arendt 1995: p.94). Additionally, knowing us as altricial humans, dependent on the other, in need of care and also care- and affection-givers, turns our relationship with the world into something very different to the relationship imposed by work, as I shall explain later.

It is true that overload of labour, like work, does not leave time, as Arendt notes, for contemplative life, for thought – the base of any truly human exercise. However, it is also true that it would be convenient to observe the movements and trends that labour creates in human beings as a survival mechanism and a care activity for oneself and others.

Bachelard obviated labour, because it is closely connected to the body, and not separated from the body and nature; because it does not become an activity that names the world separately from human beings.

Labour is thus not studied in-depth by Arendt and not at all by Bachelard. This is a pity, since from my point of view, care-taking, as part of the activity of keeping alive those who depend on us, links us to an infinite production that keeps us occupied over a very long term period. It is unproductive because it does not produce objects, but it does keep our bodies alive, connects us constantly to life and against disappearance, links us to the other who is the object of our concern, accepts the other as a vulnerable being and turns the care labour into something irreversible like action. In its repetition, it links us to the world and its avatars and prepares us much more for the field of action and creation with others.

Action

Arendt points out how "with word and action we introduce ourselves in the human world and such insertion is like a second birth... To act, in its widest sense, means having the initiative to start, as the Greek word *arkhein* shows us, or starting to move something, as the original meaning of Latin *agüere* states (Arendt 1995: p.103). Also, the action and speech are connected with the plurality, because "to live always means living among human beings, living among those who are my equals... when I enter the world, there are already others present "(p.104).

Creation as Arendt's action

I want to think about this text, with Arendt's guidance; to think of its "poetic thinking" or its "creative action" that links us to the past, present and future; that establishes a relationship between the ordinary and the extraordinary, ranging from contemplation (the thinking) to activity (the action).

I postulate that the creative process, coupled with poetic thinking may sit in the action. As we have seen, it can be placed in the sphere of work, splashing the creative process with whimsical domination and violence over matter and nature. Part of the theory of the creative process has been adopted by the creator – mostly man - with his powerful ability to use and transform the world. But this is not the perspective that interests me, since it blinds and finally destroys anyone that comes near.

There is a different concept of creation, of the creative process, close to the term of natality that Arendt uses, to plurality and to unpredictability.

> Arendt points out from action: "any further action and any new start - and we could replace this term with any new creation since they are action and start - starts a new process that will affect many... The action always produces stories, intentionally or not... But the reason why each human life tells its story and why History becomes the book of the stories of mankind, with many actors and speakers, and yet, no author, is that both are the result of the action. The real story we are committed

> to while living has no visible or invisible author, because it has not been made." (Arendt 1995: p.105)

The creative process, which can become a poetic or an artistic product, is not manufactured in the sense that Arendt interprets it, because that product is not stable, durable or objective. Only the society of each period can assign those features that become specific needs of that society, but never of the creator, or the creative action. The creator knows about the unpredictability and the fragility of the process, the plot from where he or she begins, in a magma where self and others, individuality and plurality are mixed.

> "Given that we always act in a network of relationships, the consequences of each act are unlimited, any action not only causes a chain reaction, every process is the source of unpredictable new processes... In the action, as opposed to work, it's true that we can never really know what we are doing." (Arendt 1995: p.106)

Drawing, modelling is to find a plot that changes its language as we add a trace, a mark, a signal. Each imprint results in a work and transforms its connections, rebalances or unbalances the rest. Therefore, the creative process knows of irreversibility, of the fragility of a trace and the effect of relationships.

The contingency of the beginning/at birth

Through their processes, art and creation condense in each creative act the symbolism of contingency: the accident, the unexpected and the unpredictable. The start of the creative act avoids determinism and assumes its lack of explanation, it founds without any grounds except the act of founding in itself, as Sánchez Capdeguí points out (Sánchez Capdeguí. 2009: p.68).

Therefore, every act of beginning is not in the Platonic sense of being, as a demiurge, a radical moment from which nothing becomes form. This is Bachelard's idea of creation as domination. Here the beginning is continuity and change at the same time, (following a time sequence) so each beginning is a re-beginning. As Fernando Bárcena points out,

> "the beginning is illusory: what exists is following, proceeding, linking the chain. Every beginning, every birth is nothing but an infinity renaissance, the possibility of a permanent transformation in a limited chain, which is born and dies. Among the 'still not' of what is incipient and 'not anymore' of death, there is a birth chaining." (Barcena 2003: p.106)

Many of the ideas around beginning, resound as fundamental elements of the creative process:

> "the exceptional nature of starting lies in the constituent of novelty that undermines the existing order announcing crisis, restlessness and, in the end, human reply ... The event has a great degree of ambivalence because, just as it attracts by the experience it announces, it terrifies because it breaks the automatism and the inertia of society's predictable rhythms." (Barcena 2003: p.70)

Creating is daring to start again without a rupture but pointing out a new way of being, an exercise that can explode previous structures and this is why it is an inseparable element of human freedom. To create, taking the idea of beginning an event,

> "carries us to the abyss or makes visible its disturbing presence always close and near; the event challenges our mind, it imposes a distance when facing a surprising reality ... everything comes to thinking about what does not fit, what goes against common sense, what ruins any glimpse of normality. In short, what breaks the compact unit of our experience to clear the space for the start of a new one." (Barcena 2003: p.70)

This shows the potential of the creative process through its ability to break the habit, through its thinking that diverges from lead thinking. The creative process erases the trace at the same time it points out the print, tilts towards the abyss, inviting one to the abyss, never hiding it. Creation points out the absurdity of the alien and of what is owned, opening unprecedented paths and at the same time offering a fresh look at the existing ones. Creation's glance looks back at us, at ourselves as storytellers of possible, unfinished, and provisional stories.

The importance of imagination

According to Arendt, reality is made of novelty, of unexpected events because "every event of human history reveals an unexpected landscape of actions, sufferings, and new possibilities" (Arendt 1995: p.105). Therefore,

> "only looking for a remainder of originality among the ruins, can we be able to give a response to the horrors that have taken place. The challenge of thought is to tackle the complexity of our existence in the common world and support the unpredictability and strangeness of the new." (Fuster Peiro 2009: p.51)

It leads to the need for further processes with which to search; for the creation and expression of meanings, which are the counterpart of acting.

These processes of construction of narratives are not impersonal processes, but unique embodied processes, says Fuster. These processes, such as dialogue with the events, have to be carried out by humans and cannot be based either on "simple sense" or on "pure thought", but amongst other things, on the "ability to imagine" (Fuster Peiró 2009: p.51).

The imaginative force is a means of investigating the link between humanity and the universe; the empathic imagination as a source of visionary inspiration and even as a harmonizing power of the social order. However, Arendt does not focus his idea of imagination on empathy, but rather rescues imagination as a synonym for "vision", for a lucid and penetrating glance as a synonym for "open-mindedness": imagination must guarantee enough freedom for a valid understanding, that is, to ensure a respectful representation of the unpredictable and plural structure of reality. This activity should bring us to a point of neutrality, Fuster Peiró says, that is detached but rooted in the world, from which we can face a rational development of experience without having to give up our own voice (Fuster Peiró 2009: p.54).

Imagination is the activity that makes comprehension possible: setting a distance from the given things, potentially presenting other views regarding the phenomenon and thereby enriching common belief and revealing different perspectives which compose public space (Fuster Peiró 2009: p.55). The ability to judge, therefore, has to do with meditation on and with others to reach the possibility of requesting a potential consensus.

There is only one aspect that makes action different from the creative process. Action takes place in life, in the polis, which is why it is a political act and therefore irreversible. The creative process can happen in the polis, but also in the symbolic realm of the work room, in the special space where creation takes place, which is nevertheless a laboratory of life explorations. It is a testing ground. A place for imagining. Its product confronts us with the irreversibility of creative acts in the artistic realm, which at the same time is always unfinished. It confronts us with the irreversibility of our actions in the symbolic field.

The product therefore helps us to assume error, failure and the vulnerability and fragility of our existence. It helps us to construct a story out of our pain. As Arendt says, quoting Isak Dinesen: "all sorrows can be supported if embedded in a story or if we can tell a story about them" (Dinesen cited in Arendt 2003: p.80). As Arendt wisely points out, redemption out of this misfortune of irreversibility is the power to forgive, and the remedy for unpredictability is contained in the faculty of making and keeping promises. Both remedies come together: forgiveness is linked to the past and serves to undo what has been done, while binding ourselves to promises helps to establish in the uncertain ocean of future, islands of safety (Arendt 2003: p.106). Contemplating the result of our creative process confronts us to forgive, to forgive ourselves, to forgive the world. The promise of recuperating is another act of identity and continuity that allows us to tell again our life story, knowing the fragility and the need to start over again.

Somehow, as opposed to previous statements I have exposed in this paper, there is another creation that has not to do with domain, which is not related to the instrumental, to the utilitarian in a metaphorical sense and is not related to power over others. A creation which is not domination. A creation with others, for oneself and for others, with the world, knowing the world. A creation that through its uninterrupted process which has restarted again and again, has learnt from its unpredictability and irreversibility, and has taken pleasure in so doing. This is the type of creation I want to highlight in this text, the creation that needs thought and action; contemplative life that requires solitude, and active life that requires communion with others. Reproduction, the slow and sensitive process of taking care of others, historically linked to women, has given us, in a sense, that gift: the knowledge that process does not necessarily generate finished products; that the product – in the form of beings – is never finished and does not belong to us. The labour, in the form of care and human survival, has to start over again. The joy of the labour is always short-lived, makes us humble and confronts us with the matter, the life cycle, with ourselves. It has also subjugated us as Women, of course, but using the 'epistemic privilege' of being at the margin, it allows us to see the perversion of dominance and its most cruel consequences.

There is no desire, no need, to feel pleasure in the matter that cries under the control of the worker. There is no pleasure whatsoever, if one is in no need of domination, if one lives by recognizing: re-knowing, knowing again, and opening ourselves to the dialogue between the subject and the world; taking care of ourselves with and within the world, learning how to retell it again, being conscious of the world's rhythms and ours, and being aware of our bodies, ephemeral and vulnerable.

References:

Arendt, H. (1995) *De la historia a la acción*. Barcelona, Paidós. A compilation of texts by Hannah Arendt translated into Spanish by Fina Birulés.

Arendt, H. (2003) *Conferencias sobre la filosofía política de Kant*. Barcelona, Paidos. Translated into Spanish by Carmen Corral from (1982) *Lectures on Kant's Political Philosophy*, University of Chicago Press. Chicago.

Bachelard. G. (1948) *La terre et les rêveries de la volonté* (*Earth and Reveries of Will). París, j. Corti Edition.*

De Beauvoir, S. (1949) *Deuxième sexe : Les Faits et les mythes, t. 1*, Paris, Gallimard, En español: (reed. 2006) *El segundo sexo*. Madrid, Cátedra.

Barcena, F. (2003) *El delirio de la palabras. Ensayo para una poética del comienzo*. Herder, Barcelona

Fuster Peiró, A.L. (2009) Breve topografía de una imaginación reciclada. *Revista Anthropos* (Barcelona), 3 (224), 45-56.

Sánchez Capdeguí, C. (2009) De la banalidad a la licuefacción del mal: relectura actual del totalitarismo. *Anthropos* (Barcelona), 3 (224), 62-79.

The Space Between Art Experiences and Reflective Understanding in Therapy

Mimmu Rankanen

Keywords:
Art therapy, psychophysical, embodied cognition, attachment, trauma.

Taidekokemuksen ja reflektiivisen ymmärryksen välinen terapeuttinen tila

Artikkeli käsittelee taideterapialle ominaisten toimintojen – liikkeen ja kosketuksen, katseen ja tunteen sekä ajattelun ja symbolisaation – välisten tilojen ilmenemismuotoja sekä fyysisessä taidetyöskentelyssä että kuvia katsottaessa. Aiheen käsitteellistämisessä hyödynnetään Vija Bergs Lusebrinkin (1990, 2004) systeemistä ITJ teoriaa (ETC), joka linkitetään viimeaikaiseen kehollisten kognitioiden tutkimukseen, sekä kiintymysteoriaan ja sensorimotoriseen traumateoriaan.

Teoreettista pohdintaa valaistaan kirjoittajan ohjaamaan kokemukselliseen taideterapiaryhmään osallistuneen asiakkaan kuvauksilla omasta taideterapiaprosessistaan. Asiakkaan omaa kuvausta kahden terapiaistunnon aikana tapahtuneesta kuvallisesta prosessista avataan terapeutin näkökulmasta ITJ:n avulla esitellen samalla uusi näkökulma, jossa mallia on edelleen kehitetty yksilöllisen luovan terapiaprosessin tarkastelun ja tutkimuksen välineeksi.

This paper will touch upon questions unique for arts therapies concerning the functions and implications that are manifested in the space between moving and touching, looking and feeling, thinking and symbolising, both in doing the physical artwork and reflecting the images in therapy. The aim is to conceptualize the multi-layered experience of making and viewing art in therapy by applying and further developing Vija Bergs Lusebrink's (1990, 2004) systemic theory of the Expressive Therapies Continuum, ETC.

I view and analyse the art therapy process also in the light of recent discussion and research of embodied cognitions (Damasio 2001, Folensbee 2007, Gibbs 2007, Iacobini 2008, Siegel 1999, 2007), attachment theory (Bowlby 1988) and sensory motor trauma theory (Ogden et al. 2009). The aim is to build a new perspective and coherent view of the psychophysical process, taking place in the art therapeutic relationship.

I illustrate these theoretical constructions with my client's images and written narratives of her experiences in experiential art therapy. My aim is to describe the psychophysical art therapy process in a dialogue where both the therapist's contextual view and the client's own story is heard. With this I aim to emphasise the client's role as an equal and active partner in the therapeutic working alliance, and in building theoretical understanding of the factors meaningful and effecting change in art therapy (Weinberg & Rasco 2007). These different views create space in between the experiences and conceptual understanding where new reflections can become visible.

Building bridges between creative experience and understanding

Traditional verbal therapies have largely been based on the idea that the change becomes evident because of building the narration and new story from "the top down". The hypothesis is that the change in the client's emotions and cognitions brings forth change also in other embodied levels of self. The therapeutic interventions are directed at the language of the client. Defining meanings and building reflective narratives are effective interventions - but it can be equally curative to start interventions from physical embodied experiences and move from there on towards change in understanding (Ogden et al. 2009.)

In art therapy literature the emphasis has equally been placed in developing understanding of symbolic meanings in clients' art. The varying psychophysical effects of visual and tactile art materials, creative process and imagery have often been left in a secondary position. For example McNiff (1998: p.96) has paid attention to the absence of writings focusing on the physical experiences and health-promoting effects of art-making process and perception of art. The Expressive Therapies Continuum is a developmentally structured theory, which takes into account the material and embodied levels of art therapy. It is a useful tool for perceiving how creative therapy process can connect the spaces between art experience and reflective understanding.

Expressive Therapies Continuum *Vija Bergs Lusebrink (1990, 92)*		
	Creative level	
Cognitive level	——+——	Symbolic level
Perceptual level	——+——	Affective level
Kinesthetic level	——+——	Sensory level

The structure of ETC follows individual development starting from the bottom level (Lusebrink 1990: p92). It is a contextual model of visual expression and imagery which combines knowledge of physical, sensory, emotional, cognitive, symbolic and developmental aspects to a coherent theory of art in therapy, which can be used in all psychotherapeutic paradigms (Lusebrink 1990, viii).

In what follows I look more thoroughly at each component and their role in the psychophysical space of the creative process. I focus on the therapist's point of view with respect to those implications evident in treating difficulties related to attachment and trauma, and my conceptualizations are further illuminated with my client's own story and images. The quotes throughout the paper are from the same client. She is a mother of one child, in her thirties, who at the time of participating in an experiential expressive arts therapy group was recovering from serious depression. The group I conducted was meeting for one four hour session every week and the entire process lasted 28 sessions during one year. The images and writings are chosen from my qualitative doctoral research material. All the quotations are taken from client's own written reflections after the whole therapy.

The space between moving and touching

Doing visual art there is always present the level of sensing the outside world by moving and touching. You move in the space or on the paper with your hands, brush or pencil. When you move fast, the information received is mostly kinaesthetic, sensing directions, intensity and rhythm of the movement. The art tool influences the quality of the movement as well as does the size, and horizontal or vertical direction of the paper, and if it is on the floor, table or wall. The therapist can activate, stimulate or frame the client's kinesthetic expression and help her to achieve therapeutic goals by framing or inviting the client to choose certain art materials or working positions (Rankanen 2007a). The experience of rhythm and movement can in itself be therapeutic by giving pleasure, integrating unconscious memories, repairing and activating motor memories, for example, in conditions such as Alzheimer's, strokes etc. (Lusebrink 2004).

When you slow down the movement you start to sense pressure, surface and shape by touch (Lusebrink 1990: p92). Tactile experience can be included either to touching materials outside or visceral sensation. By using tangible art materials it is possible to bridge the outer and inner experiences and become more conscious of embodied sensations. Touching different art materials stimulates the sensory level and evokes easily sensory embodied memories. Art tools limit the received sensory stimulation and can make it more bearable if the memories or emotions connected to sensory experiences are too overwhelming (Rankanen 2007b). As with exposure to anxiety provoking or traumatic stimulus it is important that the experiences stay within the manageable level and are approached gradually step by step (Litz & Salters-Pedneault 2007).

Movement and touch can evoke early implicit experiences in the present.

The kinestethic and haptic experiences are amongst the first information that is sensed by the baby while in the womb. These early childhood experiences as well as early attachment relationships are embodied and not possible to remember with declarative verbal memory. Attachment style is built before verbal and explicit memory is developed, so it is not possible to remember it cognitively. Instead, our attachment style can show in our body movements and reactions in social situations (Odgen et al. 2009: p.48-60). The way in which the first caregiver answers the baby's needs builds the attachment style between them (Bowlby 1988). The way she physically acts, uses her voice, touches and looks at the baby builds the baby's brain networks and hormonal ways to react in stressful situations (Schore 2003, Gerhard 2007). These physical reactions become automatic when the child grows.

The outer relationship between caregiver and baby becomes the person's own implicit inner ways to see herself in relation to different situations and act towards herself. The child introjects the relationships she has and they become her own inner voices. It is possible to introject both safe attachment within some relationship as insecure within another (Kanninen 2007).

> "Many members of the group carried the memory of my mother and felt familiar both in good and bad. In almost every session it was relieving to recognize those gestures and facial expressions I found jeering, neglecting and sarcastic towards me proved to be my false interpretations. After autumn I learnt to question my negative perceptions."

In art therapy these inner dialogues can manifest themselves, in addition to the therapeutic relationship, in moving and touching visible and tangible art materials.

All early childhood memories are implicit and triggered by sensory influences as are traumatic memories (Folensbee 2007: p.93-96). That is why the art therapist should be prepared and able to contain the client, and help the client to establish distance or to work thorough the varying and sometimes surprising or scaring emotions and memories that sensory information can awake. Often the fundamental work needed is to find and start to understand the connection between inner visceral and outer sensory and kinesthetic experiences.

Inner sensations and embodied experience

Focusing on sensory experiences within the art therapy process gives important information for both the therapist and client. Siegel claims that the so-called sixth sense has to do with recognizing and understanding your own body's state and the changes in it. It has not to do with sensing the outside world, but sensing the pressures and movements inside your own body, what happens in your muscles, joints and inner organs. It is essential in recognizing emotional states, as feeling angry, depressed or anxious. (Siegel 2007: p.122 &168)

Insensitivity makes it difficult to regulate emotions. Affects and emotions are embedded in the body and we learn to express and handle them only by recognizing and understanding their individual bodily forms of existence (Gibbs 2005: p.239-262). Both healthy clients suffering from life crisis and those suffering from various psychic problems are often distanced from their body. They have not learned to recognize the embodied messages or needs (Gibbs 2005: p.25-27, Rankanen 2007a: p.42-43).

Kinestethic and sensory qualities in the work with traumatic memories

Sensitising to embodied experiences is often particularly difficult for those clients who are traumatised, and it is common that they avoid painful memories by dissociating and thus escaping from too intense and overwhelming bodily sensations (Van der Kolk 2009, Ogden et al. 2009). When they are asked to concentrate on inner sensations, they either deny feeling anything or are preoccupied with overriding sensations, when traumatic sensory experience and emotions are activated in the present (Van der Kolk 2009). This makes embodied experiences unpleasant and scary and it seems better to try avoiding them all together. For effective care it is essential to confront and be exposed to avoided experiences (Johnson 2009, Litz & Salters-Pedneault 2007). Only then it is possible to learn that all varieties of sensations and emotions are safe to experience. In this process identifying the flow of sensations is essential. The embodied experience changes every moment: you do not have to remain frozen within a frightening experience (Van der Kolk 2009).

In traditional psychotherapy the explicit describing of traumatic events presumably activates implicit memories, and it shows up as unintentional physical sensations, involuntary automatic movements and negative emotions as helplessness, fear, shame and rage. Explicitly verbal therapies cannot offer restorative tools to integrate nonverbal, implicit and embodied traumatic fragments (Van der Kolk 2009).

The therapist should be aware of the risk of retraumatizing the client if the activated traumatic sensory experience is not worked through gradually and carefully enough with the client and connected to declarative explicit memory (Folensbee 2007: p.117-127). It is also essential to work first with client's capability to stay or return in her safe reflective position at the present moment before starting to work with the traumatic memories.

It is often useful to explore and strengthen the experiences and memories of safety, pleasure and competence. Working with trauma is as much remembering your own strengths, as rebuilding what was broken (Van der Kolk 2009). This all can be done in a very concrete way using those art materials, visual expressions and imageries that the client feels are enjoyable and pleasant, and that increase feelings of safety.

> *"In almost every session the work itself has brought me great happiness. While working with the most pleasant images I have also written down notes of how my hand moves and feels the materials, noticing the tactile layers of materials, how I change materials or techniques during the artwork and how I take risks or jump into the unknown."*

The space between looking and feeling

Lusebrink has contextualized the relation of visual perception and affective experience in the next level of ETC. She has paid attention to the fact that the reflective distance to the experience is small when the affective side is active - we are "in the feeling" - but when we concentrate on visual perception the reflective distance to the art experience is growing. In artwork there is normally constant flow between these two ends of the continuum (Lusebrink 1990: p.93). Most visual information is processed unconsciously and simultaneously - only a small part of the processing is conscious. Our affects have a strong impact on which of the perceptions are considered as important information and become conscious (Damasio 2001).

The more complicated feelings grow when the affects are connected with personal memories and experiences. In art therapy, colours, fluid materials, sensory and kinesthethic experiences often evoke feelings. The client describes the sources of emotional experiences:

> *"Varying sources have been affecting the evoking of feeling; the theme, warm up, happenings of the day, my relationship to the group and therapist or working with the art materials itself."* On the other hand feelings impact upon the way we work on and make choices: *"I noticed many works have started repeating the old patterns. Repetition of routines has guaranteed me safe entry to the artwork but the choices and decisions I have made later have been meaningful and important. The irritation of repeating myself has forced me towards change."*

Diving into the emotions and taking distance from them

The art therapist has a possibility to guide the client towards experiencing emotions by using the previous level of movement and touch as a bridge towards feeling. When the client is in close contact with the artwork and focusing in embodied sensations it is easier to get in touch with emotions. Working with art materials directly with the hands also increases emotional experiences.

If the emotions are instead experienced too intensely, it is possible to give more space for perceptual reflections using tools, materials or working methods, which increase structure. Consideration of aesthetic order and forms increases visual perception (Rankanen 2007b, 2007c). When the client takes distance from the image, turns it around or looks at it from different angles, it enables at the same time the possibility to take reflective distance from too overwhelming emotions:

> *"The feelings that were evoked during the artwork or connected with the image prevented me from looking at the finished picture. When I systematically concentrated on one visual element at a time the looking became easier."*

Empathy as a bridge between visual perception and emotion

The research of embodied cognitions has studied the complex relations between seeing the world outside and feeling emotions inside. There are already some studies speculating that the neural base for our capacity to empathise is dependent on a mirroring system. That gives us one explanation of how what we see is connected to our feelings. Empathy can bridge the space between eye and emotion, and this process is presumably taking place in mirror neurons, which connect the visual information with embodied experiences, postures and movements. That is why our capacity to imitate movements, body positions and facial expressions we see in others can be essential for our ability to empathise (Iacobini 2008). When we see other people's bodily expressions we feel the same in our own body and often unconsciously imitate and mirror the other person's expression to understand it in an embodied and implicit way. Siegel names this process as the seventh sense which enables us to recognize and understand other people's emotions (Siegel 2007: p.122-123, 168-169).

Cultivating empathy in the practice of art therapy

In group art therapy, imitating or following other people's ways of drawing or painting can thus be an effective method improving the group cohesiveness or creating empathy and building understanding towards others' emotions. Hintz is claiming copying as stereotyped and resistant activity (2009: p.234). However, taking into account the research of the functions of the mirroring system we can see its implications from a wider perspective. Empathy can be cultivated with somatic mirroring but more abstract forms of empathy can also be based in affective mirroring. Iacobini (2008: p.94-97) claims that only by simulating the other person's experience in our brains is it possible to deeply understand what she feels.

We can use this knowledge also as therapists and improve our ability to empathise and understand client's bodily experiences and emotions by imitating or copying her artwork in supervision. With this method it is possible to gain both implicit knowledge and at the same time reflect explicitly the ongoing art therapy process.

Copying artworks as a method of confronting and restructuring problems

Copying artworks from earlier sessions in therapy can give the client both the experience of the emotional changes that have happened and make it possible to gain a wider conscious perspective and reflective understanding. It is an especially useful method when returning to and working through a negatively charged image later in therapy. The exposure to objects of emotional and behavioural avoidance and gaining mastery experiences is a very important factor influencing the effectiveness of all psychotherapies (Clinton et al. 2007, Weinberg & Rasco 2007).

> *"Now later on I see as most important those images where I have caught a feeling and let myself experience it while working. The most rewarding feelings have come when I have faced painful thoughts, worked with problems and tried to solve conflicts during the artwork."*

When working with images connected to strong negative emotions it is essential not to dive into the emotions evoked but to copy the artwork staying consciously in a reflective state of mind. The therapeutic change is greatest when the emotional stress is moderate (Clinton et al. 2007). Paying careful attention to the visual elements of the artwork and writing down all explicit thoughts, sensations and feelings while copying alleviates it. At a suitable point the client can work on freely as she wishes. Often it is possible to gain remarkable insights through this process. It can give a strong feeling of controlling one's own experiences and reactions which is again an important common factor (Clinton et al. 2007, Weinberg & Rasco 2007).

The space between thinking and symbolising

Thinking as well as symbolising includes previous levels of movement, touch, seeing and feeling. They develop latest in childhood and are partly dependent on abilities developed earlier. Thinking and symbolising are not only verbal processes but include visual thinking, visual problem-solving and an implicit understanding of embodied meanings. Even if the embodied part of the construction is not conscious the whole body is actively working in constructing meanings and understanding (Gibbs 2007: p.40). From recent studies it is possible to make conclusions that thinking is not happening in our brains separated from body, but our movements and gestures precede and help us to create new verbal and constructive thinking (Iacobini 2008, Gibbs 2007). Our affects and emotions effect the perceptions that become conscious and guide our reasoning and thinking (Damasio 2001). This can be evident in art therapy when noticing that images can change their meanings depending on the emotional state in which one perceives them.

Symbolising and creating meanings is enhanced by feelings evoked during the art-making process. Meanings can also be connected to touch and other body sensations long before verbalising (Gibbs 2007: p.86-90). The physical art-making process can contain personal meanings or memories different from or even conflicting with the ones evoked when looking at the art object (Rankanen 2007b). By using art in thinking and solving problems we can connect symbolic meanings and construct a coherent view of complicated and many-sided life experiences and social relationships.

The client's story

This art process happened during two four-hour experiential expressive arts therapy group sessions that followed each other (17th and 18th of a total of 28 sessions). The client was asked to take with her some photos she wanted to work with in therapy. The first session gives an example of "top to down" art therapy process where the client attempts to control difficult feelings with cognitive thinking, planning and visual structuring. The emotions are connected with the traumatic moments of separation from mother, which have been recurring throughout the client's childhood.

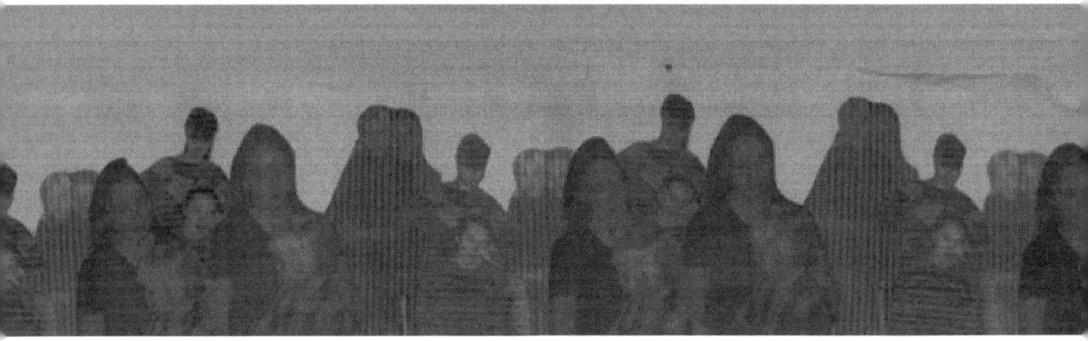

1. *"I was full of expectations when we started to work with the photos. I had chosen photos from those recurring moments when my mother went away and left me. I felt the images to be extremely painful in an uncontrollable way. Beforehand I explained to myself that I would overcome the fear and grief of my childhood at once."* Figure 1

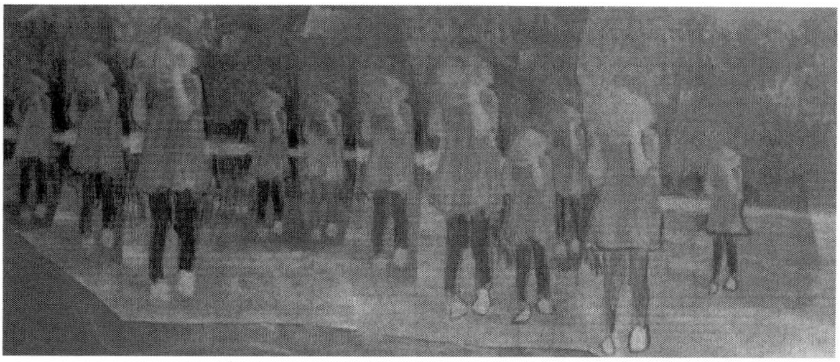

Figure 2

2. *"Cutting the copies of the photos and organizing them on paper felt both slow and burdensome work. I tried to make the work easier with ornaments. I tried to replace the feeling of pain by working hard. But the work was never finished. My notebook was left empty without a word."*

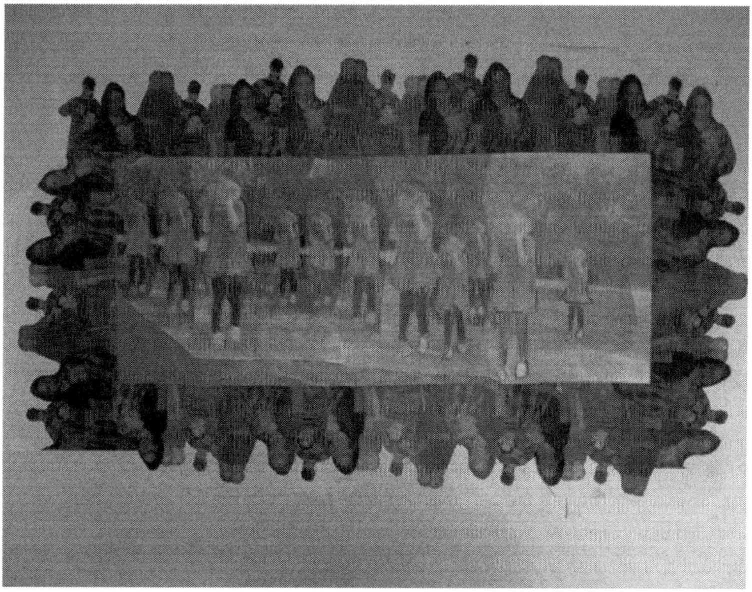

Figure 3

3. "When we looked at the image M said it looks like a repeating experience of horror and those words remained echoing in my mind. Later when I looked at the image I saw its deceitful beauty and decorations but at the same time felt its heavy feeling. Melancholy filled my mind."

The process continues in the next four-hour session. The client decides to work on with the same photo that contains painful and traumatic memories. This time she engages in creative restructuring by building safe and soothing experience for herself instead of repeating the traumatic memories. She is able to let go of too restrictive cognitive planning and control, and engages in an intuitive creative process. She restructures the traumatic emotional experience with spontaneous artwork. Building embodied sensory - not explicitly cognitive - experience of trust and care opens up the possibility to reframe earlier experiences and makes it possible to challenge the repeating of the traumatic experience.

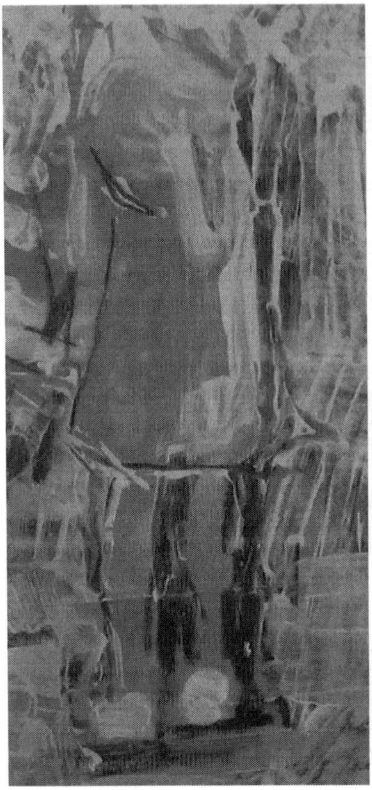

Figure 4

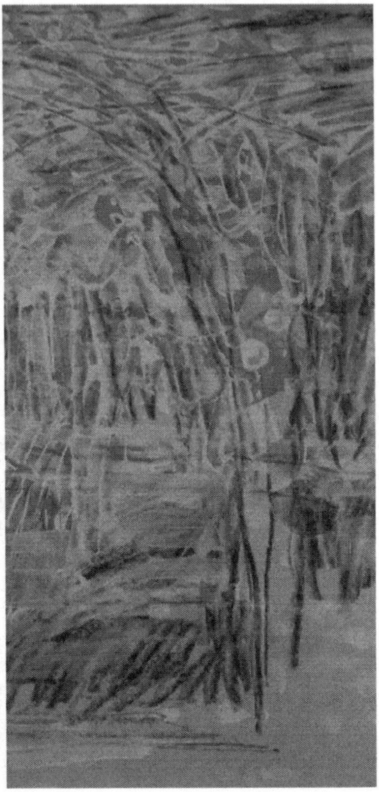

Figure 5

4. " Luckily I could continue working in the next session. I wanted to stay with the same theme and I had with me the same photo as on the previous week. I had again been planning a manuscript for what I wanted to do. But this time it was so caring and soothing that following it was not violent to my feelings. I would place the painful image of myself as a child to the garden with another image of me as an adult."

5. "I didn't have any plans how to make the image or what it could look like. I started to work very fast, as if I was afraid that the threads I followed would disappear. And still, at the same time, I was very confident and joyful. As a base for the image I used orange and yellow cardboard, which I tapped full of white dots with my fingers."

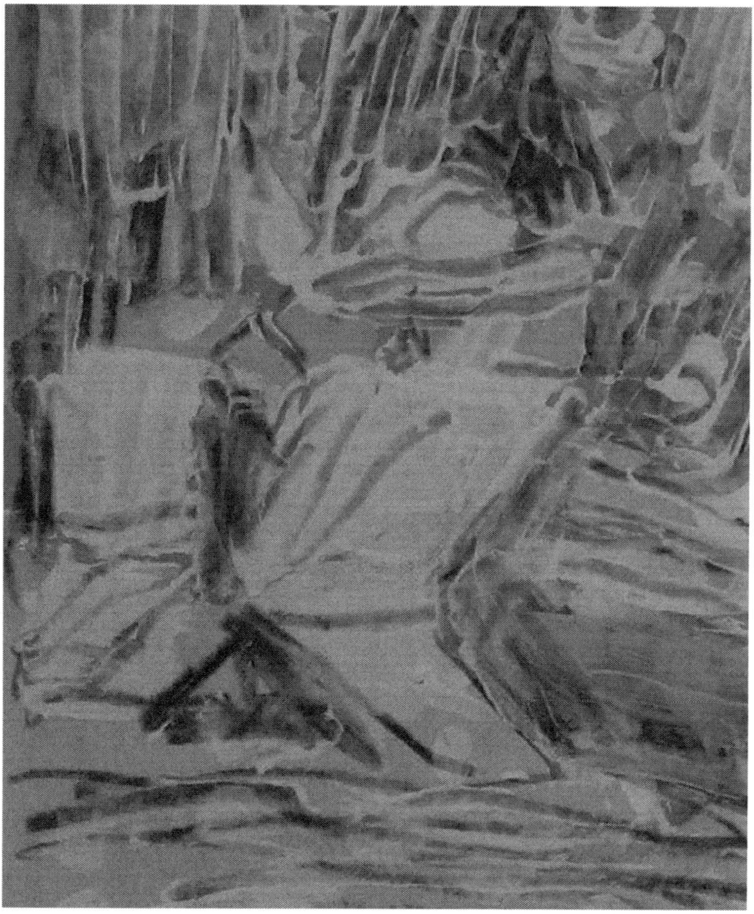

Figure 6

6. "I didn't have time to copy the photo of the adult me. It made the working more free and relaxed. In the end I spontaneously added a sunhat, an open book and a chair to the otherwise finished garden. I had a strong and encouraging sense of Mother's presence through the whole working. When I added the symbols to the image she became real."

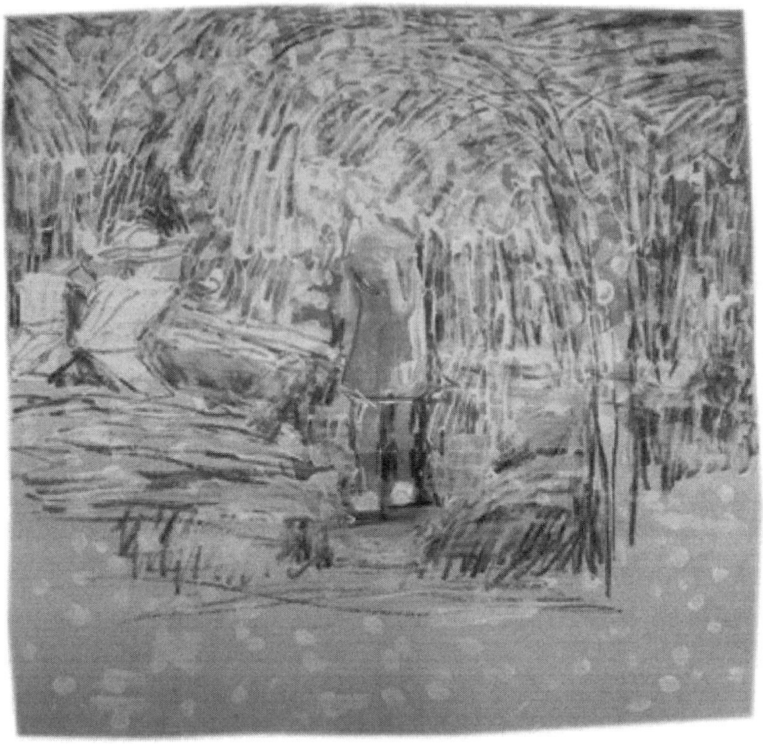

Figure 7

7. "The little me from the photo stands in the middle of the white, yellow and orange light sparkling everywhere. On top of the white fingerprints I drew black lines, which gives direction to the landscape and curves around the girl. The colours are weirdly bright. The lines of the drawing are strong and fast. I named the painting 'Under the same tree'. It turned out to be a treasure for me."

Understanding the individual creative process

The creative process can connect all the previous spaces and it can be experienced as a flow or as a synthesis between different levels (Lusebrink 1990, 2004). It is fundamentally not controllable but surprising. However, it is possible to influence it with art materials and methods chosen. A therapist can set realistic goals for each unique client by taking into account where the blocks of the creative therapy process are situated and which are spaces where the connections should be repaired. Therefore I argue ETC model can be further developed in the following way:

Creative Process	
Cognitive processes Problem solving, conceptual thinking, planning	Symbolic processes Meanings, metaphors
Visual perception Shape, colour, size, distance	Emotions Positive, negative
Movement Rhythm, speed, direction	Tactile experiences Outer, inner

By opening the space between these different levels, it is possible for a therapist to draw a map, and use it as a tool for structuring and understanding the proceeding of an individual art therapy process.

When looking at my client's story and images (1. – 2.), we can see she began the process from the cognitive level trying to avoid the painful emotion by thinking and planning carefully the picture's visual structure, shapes, sizes and distances where she placed the photocopy images. When she perceived the picture (3.), she created a connection between looking and feeling and experienced the avoided emotion. In the following session (phase 4.), there has happened a change in her inner dialogue, and the child's pain and sorrow in her that has been avoided and not accepted, is now looked after and caressed. She is in contact with her emotional experiences and both inner and outer sensations (5.), which enables the spontaneous creative flow and movement (Phase 6.). She feels safe and trusting and can express the emotions with relaxed movements and creates meaningful symbols. The process ends (7.) with coherent experience of integration and synthesis between all the levels.

Blocks of the creative therapy process

In all the psychotherapies blocks and ruptures in the process and therapists' ability to repair them are central for successful treatments (Ruiz-Cordell & Safran 2007). The blocks manifest in different ways depending on client and her stage of change. In the art therapy process the ruptures or resistances are not only experienced in the therapeutic relationship but also in these different levels of the creative process itself. It is possible that the blocks are not manifested at a single level but in the undeveloped or blocked connection between two or more levels.

My client was at times blocked off from emotional experiences. When there was not enough energy, courage or trust to focus on present emotions, the process could be directed in perceptual experiences:

> *"Sometimes I fidgeted from routines towards presence by observing the environment. I wrote or sketched and observations worked as a life buoy, but were not enough for creating a meaningful work. I did not face the crisis and that is why there has been no (possibility for) solution either. I am embarrassed by those works that have not reached the poignancy of the present moment. In part I had worked with painful or emotional issues and I respect that. Still the emotions were not faced sensing the present experience."*

At other times she could avoid feelings by staying in cognitive space. Her attempt to avoid emotions was at the same time blocking the creative process: *"The artwork was heavy, laborious and fruitless when I have either worked against my emotions or neglecting them."* When the client was not feeling safe or did not have trust enough it was difficult to enter the spontaneous creative process and let go of too restrictive cognitive controlling or planning.

In enabling the creative therapeutic process for my client, it seemed crucial to find both a safe space and suitable art methods for building bridges between the spaces of explicit cognitive planning and implicit bottom level experiences:

> *"When I stared at the artwork from thinking and writing about my problem, the perfectionist in me awoke and froze me. I was afraid my incapability would be revealed to others and that was why I started doing spontaneous mono prints. I worked fast and without a plan. I felt my pulse rate speeding up and felt great. The images did not look good, but the free and spontaneous technique was very different from my normal habits. I felt very courageous. I managed to change the pressure of conscious thinking into a satisfactory creative work and continue working in spite of panic and fright."*

Conclusions

In psychotherapy as well as art therapy too intense concentration in verbal thinking and the client's stories can leave the therapy superficial. It can make us underestimate the therapeutic power of embodied sensory, motoric or visual experiences, which can have a direct effect upon our self-regulation of stress and immune functions (Siegel 2009). In art therapy it is an important element of cure to integrate these different flows of information and knowledge systems and thus enable the building of coherent - not chaotic - and controllable enough experience of self in the world. It becomes possible when we integrate our implicit embodied experiences and memories with our explicit reflective knowledge.

I claim that the embodied creative work with varying art materials, and the movements, sensations, perceptions, emotions and cognitions they activate or evoke are important and effective therapeutic factors if the art therapist has a coherent theory with which to contextualize the process and on which to base the methods used in art therapy. Understanding the theoretical construction and relationships of these spaces gives us clarity and provides tools for using the art process effectively in therapy.

References

Bowlby, J. (1988) *A Secure Base: Parent-child attachment and healthy human development.* New York, Basic Books.

Clinton, D., Gierlach, E., Zack, S., Beutler, L., and Castonguay, L. (2007) Toward the Integration of Technical Interventions, Relationship Factors, and Participants Variables. In: Hoffman, S. and Weinberger, J. (eds.) *The Art and Science of Psychotherapy.* New York, Routledge, pp.130-153.

Damasio, A. (1994) *Descartes Error. Emotion, Reason and the Human brain.* Putnam Publishing, New York.

Folensbee, R. W. (2007) *The Neuroscience of Psychological Therapies.* Cambridge, Cambridge University Press.

Gerhard, S. (2004) *Why love matters. How affection shapes a baby's brain.* East Sussex, Routledge.

Gibbs, R. (2005 [reprinted 2007]) *Embodiment and Cognitive Science.* Cambridge, Cambridge University Press.

Hinz, L. (2009) *Expressive Therapies Continuum. A Framework for Using Art in Therapy.* New York, Routledge.

Iacobini, M. (2008) *Mirroring People, The New Science of How We Connect With Others.* Farrar, Straus and Giroux, New York.

Johnson, D. R. (2009) Examining underlying Paradigms in the creative arts therapies of trauma. *Arts in Psychotherapy,* 36, 114-120.

Kanninen, K. (2007) Dialogisen mielen rakentuminen varhaisessa vuorovaikutuksessa. In: Lindeman, M., Hokkanen, L.& Punamäki, R-L. (eds.) *Hermoverkot, mielenterveys ja psykoterapia.* Psykologien kustannus, pp.72-83.

Litz, B. & Salters-Pedneault, K. (2007) The Art of Evidence-Based Treatment of Trauma Survivors. In: Hoffman, S. & Weinberger, J. (eds.) *The Art and Science of Psychotherapy.* New York, Routledge, pp. 211-230.

Lusebrink, V. (1990) *Imagery and Visual Expression in Therapy.* New York, Plenum Press.

Lusebrink, V. (2004) Art therapy and the brain: An Attempt to Understand the Underlying Processes of Art Expression in Therapy. *Art Therapy: Journal of the American Art Therapy Association,* 21(3), 125-135.

McNiff, S. (1998) *Art-based research.* Philadelphia, Jessica Kingsley Publishers.

Ogden, P., Minton, K., & Pain C. (2009) *Trauma ja keho. Sensorimotorinen psykoterapia.* Oulu: Traumaterapiakeskus. Translated by Pekkarinen, I. from: *Trauma and the Body.* (2006). New York, W.W. Norton & Company, Inc.

Rankanen, M. (2006) Luonnoksia kuvataideterapian, terapeuttisen kuvantekemisen ja kuvataideopetuksen suhteista. (Sketches of the proportions of art therapy, therapeutic art and art education) In:

Kettunen, K., Hiltunen M., Laitinen S. and Rastas M. (eds.) *Kuvien keskellä.* Keuruu: Like, pp189-199.

Rankanen, M. (2007a) Taideterapiassa vaikuttavia ydinprosesseja. In: Rankanen, M., Hentinen, H. & Mantere, M. (eds.) *Taideterapian perusteet.* ("The Principles of Art Therapy") Hämeenlinna: Duodecim, pp.34–49.

Rankanen, M. (2007b) Kuvataiteen erityispiirteet terapian jäsentäjinä. In: Rankanen, M., Hentinen, H. & Mantere, M. (eds.) *Taideterapian perusteet.* Hämeenlinna: Duodecim, pp.64–89.

Rankanen, M. (2007c) Taidetyöskentely. In: Rankanen, M., Hentinen, H. & Mantere, M. (eds.) *Taideterapian perusteet.* Hämeenlinna: Duodecim, pp.112–126.

Rankanen, M. (2009) Läsnäolon, kohtaamisen ja oivalluksen kuvia. (Images of presence, contact and insight) *STYLUS* 2/2009, 8-9.

Ruiz-Cordell, K. & Safran, J. (2007) Alliance Ruptures. Theory, Research and Practice. In: Hoffman, S. & Weinberger, J. (eds.) *The Art and Science of Psychotherapy.* New York, Routledge, pp. 155 – 170.

Schore, A. (2003) *Affect Dysregulation and Disorders of the Self.* New York, Norton.

Siegel, D. (1999) *The Developing Mind: How Relationships and the Brain Interact to Who We Are.* New York,Guildford Press.

Siegel, D. (2007) *The Mindful Brain: Reflection and Attunement in the Cultivation of Well-Being.* New York, W. W. Norton & Company.

Siegel, D. (2009) Vuorovaikutteisen neurobiologian näkökulma. In: Ogden, P., Minton, K. & Pain, C. *Trauma ja keho. Sensorimotorinen psykoterapia.* Oulu: Traumaterapiakeskus. Translated by Pekkarinen, I. from: *Trauma and the Body* (2006) New York, W.W. Norton & Company, Inc., pp.xv – xviii.

Van der Kolk, B. (2009) Esipuhe. In: Ogden, P., Minton, K., & Pain, C. *Trauma ja keho. Sensorimotorinen psykoterapia.* Oulu: Traumaterapiakeskus. Translated by Pekkarinen, I. from: *Trauma and the Body* (2006) New York, W.W. Norton & Company, Inc. pp.xix - xxviii

Weinberg, J. & Rasco, C. (2007) Empirically Supported Common Factors. In: Hoffman, S. & Weinberger, J. (eds.) *The Art and Science of Psychotherapy.* New York, Routledge, pp.103–129.

Cultivating the Habit of Art in Therapy

Malcolm Ross

> "It seems to me pleasing that writers of another age, and from another civilization... should arrive at conclusions... traceable in what constitutes arguably the greatest intellectual tradition of the West... They shared this vital sense of the contingent nature of things." (McGilchrist 1982: p.239-240)

In this paper I argue that creativity in the arts may be usefully modelled upon the natural, 'creative' cycle of the seasons. More particularly I adopt the ancient Chinese Taoist tradition of the five elements – also known as the five phases of change. That change is the natural condition of human experience seems incontrovertible: handling change at the biological level is accounted for in evolutionary theory in terms of the twin principles of 'adaptation' and 'natural selection'. To survive and develop successfully in an uncertain environment, the human species, like all other forms of life, has had to learn to adapt; at the same time, so evolutionary theory tells us, our survival has been bound up with physical changes, including the growth in size and change in structure of the brain, which has made us 'fitter' for reproductive success than other species with whom we are in competition. Chinese Taoist philosophy positions us in dynamic interaction with the natural environment, sharing its constituent elements and subject to the flow of its energies. Its central regulatory idea is that of the balance and the reconciliation of opposites: of an essentially harmonious set of relationships, regularly disturbed but just as regularly re-established. I shall argue that there is much to be gained by conceiving of creativity in the arts as a process of 'illumination' – rather than, as has been the more familiar case with us, as a series of discrete, 'problem-solving' projects managed upon the mechanical model of in-put and out-put. Where our own tradition favours a linear, product-oriented configuration, the model I am proposing is cyclical and revelatory.

Rom Harré and the Identity Project

In modelling the arts curriculum in education I have for many years used the two-dimensional matrix developed by Rom Harré in his book *Personal Being* (1983) for what he calls 'the identity project'. Harré understands the process of personal development as essentially 'expressive'. His model of personal being has two dimensions: *public-private* and *individual-collective*. Since language is the principal cultural agency in the development of identity he tracks the infant's acquisition of language skills through the model's four phases:

1. **Conventionalization**: The infant is immersed in a language environment from birth and, given a brain hard-wired for language acquisition and use, immediately embarks upon distinguishing I from It and Thou: marking the beginnings of two complementary conversations with the world. This is largely effected interactively with the mother
2. **Appropriation**: There is a gradual shift in the infant's perception from language as an expressive environment to language as an expressive medium – more particularly, from language as 'other' to language as an extension of the self. Once again, the primary partner in what becomes language play is the mother.
3. **Transformation**: With a shared expressive language with which to express themselves, infants graduate to selective reception and creative transformation – language becomes a vehicle of personal meaning – i.e., symbolic of identity.
4. **Publication**: The destination of language in action is inter-personal communication and collaboration. Through language that modulates between the transactional and the expressive as occasion requires, the infant becomes established as a member of a language-using community. Harré's model looks like this:

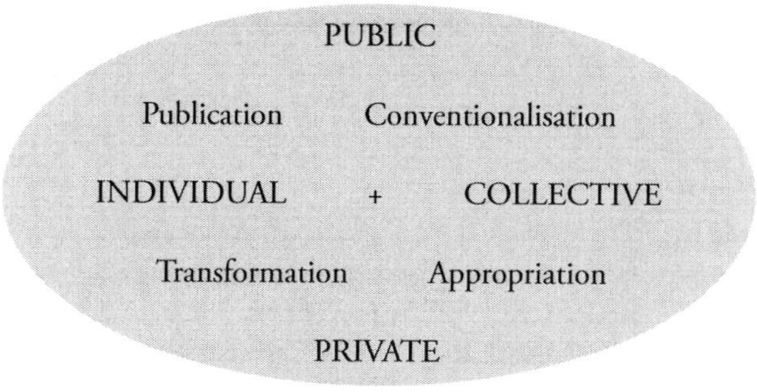

My model of the arts curriculum (Ross et al. 1993) was an adaptation of what seemed an essentially creative schema to the creative process in the arts. It was intended to provide a basis for curriculum planning and an effective, participatory pedagogy, and also to serve as a framework for systematic assessment – all of which were thought to be problematic at the time of the research. The four phases of the arts curriculum were understood as a cycle rather than as a circle.

1. **Conventionalization**: The student inherits a culture and through immersion within it learns its codes and conventions. Where, for whatever reason, the student is felt to lack a rich enough cultural stock, including a command of technical skills, then remedial steps are taken to address this deficiency. Creativity in the arts does not exist in a vacuum.
2. **Appropriation**: The next phase sees the students finding their own voices, developing their own tastes and preferences, both as makers and receivers of the arts. It is a question of making the culture their own – of feeling at home in it and confident in answering their own personal expressive impulses.
3. **Transformation**: Depending upon those tastes and inclinations, the developing artist will forge a practice of symbol-making and symbol-use suited to themselves as they seek to explore and express personal emotional meaning through the arts.
4. **Publication**: The impulse of artistic expression is understood to issue in a social event of sharing and mutual encountering, where gifts are exchanged and measure taken of the work done. The moment of publication is as much sought after as the moment of creative inspiration.

A fully participatory pedagogy has the teacher actively engaged at every phase of the process. An adequate system of appraisal will cover all four phases of a student's creativity – and, in keeping with the dialogical nature of the project, will be likely to aim at negotiation and consensus. My research colleagues and I appropriated Harré's description: for us, creativity in the arts was an 'identity project'. This was the link we made to the traditional notion, long beloved of arts teachers, that arts education was about personal growth and emotional development (Ross 1978). The model became synonymous with 'the intelligence of feeling' (Wikin 1974).

Five Elements Theory

My introduction to Chinese Five Element Theory came courtesy of my acupuncturist Donna Ashton. I quickly saw a powerful correspondence with Harré and began trying to integrate them. Since the Chinese model was clearly about creativity in the wider contexts of nature and health, and, as I subsequently discovered, was also known as the Five Phases of Change, such a project didn't seem entirely outlandish.

Five Element Theory proposes that we are part of a pervasive and continuing system of energies (*chi*) influencing processes of growth and decay in the world. Like all living things we are composed of five elements: Earth, Fire, Metal, Water, Wood. Each element is a force field of energy and exerts its own particular influence. When we are healthy, these energies are flowing together through the body linking us with the life force flowing through the world. When these energies become blocked or unbalanced, then we become sick, in body, mind or spirit. Healing is a matter of restoring flow or balance by specified techniques – in the case of acupuncture by the judicious placing of needles at key points along the energy channels (known as 'meridians'). Learning to keep healthy and creative is a matter of maintaining the flow and balance of one's vital forces.

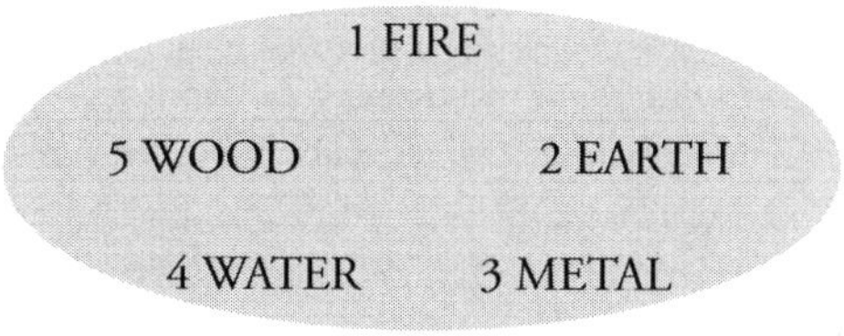

Each of the Five Elements is identified by a profile of corresponding special features and influences. Each has its own colour, its material associations, physical characteristics, associated season and characteristic emotion.

Metal	White	Gold, Tin	Radiation	Dry	Autumn	Grief
Water	Blue	Rain, Sea	Inundation	Cold	Winter	Fear
Wood	Green	Vegetation	Flower and Fall	Wind	Spring	Rage
Fire	Red	Fire	Explosion	Heat	Summer	Joy & Love
Earth	Yellow	Soil	Fertility	Damp	Late Summer	Empathy

Five Element Theory holds that as individuals we are governed by one (sometimes two) key element (s). My element is Fire for instance, Donna's is Water. In treating her patient the acupuncturist takes this typical factor into account with a view to restoring the special harmonies appropriate to it. Assessing an individual's element is difficult for the uninitiated: it is a professional skill. It has nothing to do with date of birth. There is a powerful connection between personality and the influence of bodily organs. Here is a simplified account:

	Yin	*Yang*			
Metal	Lungs	Large Intestine	Inspiring	Conservative	Judgement
Water	Kidneys	Bladder	Wise	Commitment	Courage
Wood	Liver	Gallblader	Assertive	Creative	Hope
Fire	Heart	Small Intestine	Sociable	Passionate	Affection
Earth	Spleen	Stomach	Nurturing	Compassionate	Grounded

The twin principles of Yin Yang account for the contrary inclinations we all have towards inwardness, solitariness and reflection on the one hand, and being outgoing, sociable and expressive on the other (a rough equivalent would be the introversion-extraversion distinction). We are each subject to sunshine and shadow.

The dynamic nature of the theory is best expressed as a double tendency: on the one hand toward nourishing and on the other toward resisting (even destroying). The nourishing tendency of the cycle is called *Sheng*; the challenging tendency is called *Ke* (pronounced Ko). These two tendencies bring the five elements into a range of different, complementary relationships. For example, Earth nourishes Metal which in turn nourishes Water. A weakness or malfunction in a particular element, picked up in the process of diagnosis or assessment, raises questions for the healing practitioner about lack of nourishment and lack of resistance. Problems with nourishment, in the Water element for instance, might indicate a lack of support from Metal. Similarly, over-stimulation can also lead to exhaustion and imbalance, perhaps suggesting a failure in the controlling system: treating exhausted or over-active Metal might mean strengthening the impact of Fire within the patient.

Sheng (Nourishing)	*Ke* (Controlling)
Earth > METAL > Water	Wood < METAL < Fire
Metal > WATER > Wood	Fire < WATER < Earth
Water > WOOD > Fire	Earth < WOOD < Metal
Wood > FIRE > Earth	Metal < FIRE < Water
Fire > EARTH > Metal	Water < EARTH < Wood

The Syncretic Model of creativity in the arts

Donna and I developed what we came to call the Syncretic Model of Creativity in the Arts, bringing Harré and Five Element Theory together, with Donna herself placing the element of Earth at the centre in accordance with the oldest of the Chinese representations, thereby adding a major new factor to the earlier formulation. It gradually became clear to me as we worked on it that the new model was vastly richer in its implications than the original one based on Harré, due to its inherently *dynamic* character – as explained above. Here is the Syncretic Model as we created it.

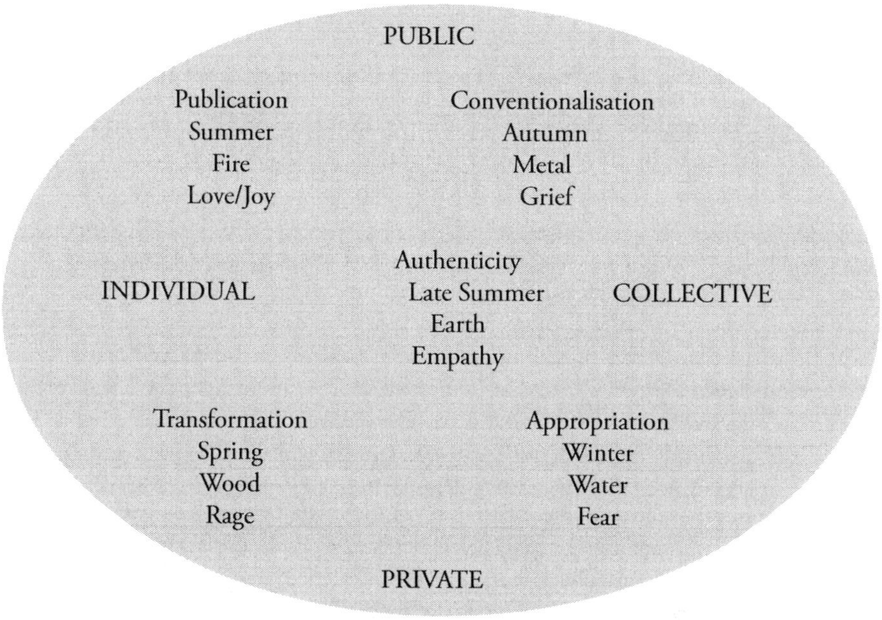

At the centre of the creative cycle in the arts, the Earth phase is the artist's authenticity. This remains the taproot to the integrity of the whole project. The model shows this central phase overlapping each of the other three, making its influence continuous and pervasive. Whatever imperils authenticity imperils the whole creative project. Earth is also the seat of empathy, and empathy in the aesthetic domain equates to the intelligence of feeling. The Metal phase represents the culture within which the creative project is situated. It represents the storehouse of tradition and wisdom, and supplies the artist's inspiration. It also holds the promise of survival, as the completed work, at the end of the cycle, exerts its influence for change. The Water phase sees the artist confront the risks of creativity and the challenge to make their own mark, make their own voice heard. At Wood the creative force is given its head and drives all before it in its 'rage' to be. Fire follows, with its praise and with its celebration, as the individual creator rejoins the community with their gift to share. Earth has been constant throughout the process but has its own special moment as the artist confronts their own work, and puts it to the toughest test of all: authenticity. Finally comes the Metal phase of public judgement, when the guardians have their say and the cycle starts again.

The task of the arts teacher and arts therapist, as I understand their distinctive but complementary work, is to be present with their student, client or patient at every phase of the cycle, checking its strength or ministering to its weakness, maintaining or restoring balance and flow so the project may achieve its promise. And that project, that promise, as I see it, is expressive, is purely and simply the making or the receiving of the symbol that answers the individual's desire, that supplies the individual's essentially transcendent yearning for 'illumination' – meaning, knowing. We are still talking about identity. It does so, I want to suggest, because thinking in metaphors, thinking in presentational symbols, thinking in images, thinking in feeling, causes new feeling structures to form in the brain, thus allowing feelings to be unblocked, rebalanced, elaborated and transformed. So the intelligence of feeling grows. I present a detailed account of what a participatory practice in arts education and therapy might look like, in my new book, *Cultivating the Arts in Education and Therapy* (2011). Here is Gadamer, on the symbol in art:

> "The symbolic representation accomplished in art does not have to depend directly on what is already given. On the contrary, it is characteristic of art that what is represented, whether it is rich or poor in connotations or has none whatsoever, calls us to dwell upon it and to give our assent in an act of recognition… Art is only encountered in a form that resists conceptualisation. Great art shakes us because we are always unprepared and defenceless when exposed to the overpowering impact of a compelling work. Thus the essence of the symbolic lies precisely in the fact that it is not related to an ultimate meaning that could be recuperated in intellectual terms. The symbol preserves its meaning within itself." (Gadamer 1986: p.43)

Iain McGilchrist, in his book *The Master and his Emissary* (2010), makes much of the way we in the West have come to allow the left hemisphere of the brain to ride roughshod over the right hemisphere, giving us an altogether unbalanced approach to life and the world we live in. He claims that the right brain is actually our species' default brain – with its characteristic inclination towards a broad, cohesive, rounded approach to life, whereas the left brain, particularly aggressive and dominant since the Age of Enlightenment in the 18th century, inclines towards analysis, calculation, the literal and the particular. Left brain deals in referential and discursive symbols, whereas the right brain handles experience through presentational symbols (see Langer 1967), metaphor and myth. Left brain is dominated by the intelligence of individual reason; right brain prefers the intelligence of mutual feeling. As I see it, the beauty of the Syncretic Model, where arts teachers and therapists are concerned, is that it reconciles the two hemispheres in an holistic endeavour: where the individual elements, individually considered, might be seen to operate largely under the influence of the left brain, the dynamic character of the model (its *Sheng* and *Ke* cycles) are a perfect illustration of right brain activity, nourishing and challenging through a complex of inter-elemental relationships. In an earlier book, from which I quote at the top of this paper, McGilchrist (1982) anticipates my invocation of the ancient Chinese writers of the Tao, linking them to the Greek philosopher Heraclitus and with what he calls 'the great sceptical humanist writers during the period of four or five hundred years from which most of what we study as literature derives.' In researching for my own book (2011) I have found a growing interest among writers on creativity in what can be learned from the East. In my book I try to make the case for cultivating the habit of art as therapy.

References

Gadamer, H-G. (1986) *The Relevance of the Beautiful and Other Essays.* Cambridge: Cambridge University Press

Harré, R. (1983) *Personal Being: A Theory for Individual Psychology.* Oxford: Basil Blackwell Publisher Ltd

Langer, S. K. (1967) *Philosophy in a New Key.* Cambridge Massachusetts: Harvard University Press

McGilchrist, I. (1982) *Against Criticism.* London: Faber and Faber Limited

McGilchrist, I. (2010) *The Master and His Emissary.* New Haven and London: Yale University Press

Ross, M. (1978) *The Creative Arts.* London: Heinemann Educational Books Ltd

Ross, M., Radnor, H., Mitchell, S.& Bierton, K. (Eds.) (1993) *Assessing Achievement in the Arts*, Buckingham: Open University Press.

Ross, M. (2011) *Cultivating the Arts in Education and Therapy.* London: Routledge

Witkin, R. W. (1974) *The Intelligence of Feeling.* London: Heinemann Educational Books

Creating Social Bonds and Creating the Self in the Transitional Space of Dance-Rhythm Therapy

France Schott-Billmann

(Translated from French by Eleanor Hendriks)

Création du lien social et création de soi dans l'aire transitionnelle en danse-rythme thérapie.

Résumé:

Le danse-rythme-thérapeute s'inspire des principes rythmiques qui sous-tendent les jeux mère-enfant dans l'aire transitionnelle. En effet, on peut établir un parallèle entre l'objectif du thérapeute qui cherche à libérer le patient psychotique de l'état de fusion-confusion dans lequel « il n'y a pas d'autre », et celui de la mère qui amène l'enfant à la capacité de se relier à l'autre humain, de façon équilibrée, c'est-à-dire de façon ni trop proche (trop de fusion, c'est à dire l'envahissement) ni trop éloignée (trop de séparation, c'est à dire isolement, abandon et solitude).

Le rythme du va et vient ou balancement (pensons au bercement) est un mouvement bipolaire qui crée deux espaces et deux temps. Il contient donc un pouvoir de différenciation que le thérapeute va exploiter de différentes façons. Le va-et-vient du rythme qui fait balancer le corps permet d'articuler ses deux moitiés ce qui a pour effet de l'unifier, de libérer le patient du fantasme de morcellement. Mais le va-et-vient du rythme sera utilisé aussi pour construire un balancement dans la relation entre patient et thérapeute, chacun disposant en alternance d'un temps identique pour s'exprimer par la voix et le mouvement. Un dialogue rythmique s'instaure, où émerge progressivement pour le patient, la notion d'altérité : le thérapeute n'est pas lui, ils sont différents, ce qui, précisément, permet l'échange et le partage.

The clinical position of the therapist working with psychotic patients is not unlike the role of the mother in relation to her child. The individual, a patient in the first case and a child in the other, is accompanied along a course which liberates him or her from the fusional or symbiotic relationship he or she has with the *other*. In this symbiotic state, interior and exterior, the self and the *other*, the imaginary and the real are indistinguishable and the individual's capacity to differentiate and to organize interpersonal relations is hindered. Since this fusion confuses the boundaries between individuals, it is antithetical to building human relationships. The capacity to relate to others depends on the exteriorization of the *other*. The *other* must be recognized as other-than-self and its alterity must be understood as radically differentiating it from the self. The very desire to bond with another individual is made possible by one's feelings of distinctness and intrapsychic independence. True human bonds do not imprison individuals; rather they act like bridges joining separate individuals.

The capacity to differentiate is at the origin of human relationships. It also enables coherent thinking and provides access to the symbolic function (Levis-Strauss 1965; Freud 1981), that is to say, the expression of representations of the self using verbal and non-verbal forms, such as words, graphic productions, gestures and sounds.

This prodigious work, accomplished by the mother with her child, renewed every generation, is accomplished progressively through a transition between symbiosis, where the infant is attached to the mother, part of her body and felt to be one with her, and the discovery that they are in fact two beings separated by their alterity and that one is not the other.

Inspired by this ancestral know-how, the dance-rhythm therapist also carefully arranges a transition for the patient by establishing a space for play, what Winnicott (1971: p.11) precisely called an "intermediary area" or "potential space" which opens *play* in the symbiotic fusion. It allows for the discovery of the notion of alterity, or otherness, at the heart of the therapist-patient duo as it does in the mother-infant dyad. In dance-rhythm therapy, the transitional space is rhythmic. It is through sharing a common rhythm with the therapist that the patient will be able to discover the pleasure of social relationships that far from imprisoning, is liberating.

1. Rhythm: the transition between nature and culture

In humanizing her child, the mother uses an essential tool – rhythm. Infants are very sensitive to the maternal voice which they learn to recognize in the womb. The maternal voice reaches the fetus filtered by the liquid envelope surrounding it, and is heard along with, and accentuated by, the mother's heartbeat and breathing. These elements, altogether, form the rhythmic background for all of the fetus's intrauterine sensorial-motor experiences. Everything that reaches it from the outside, noises and familiar voices, is inscribed on this internal canvas.

According to Françoise Dolto, rhythm is pre-linguistic, "a basic pre-temporo-spatial signifier, and therefore fetal" (Dolto 1982: p.147). Indeed, the genius of motherhood is exactly its use of natural rhythms to draw the infant into the culture, that is to say, toward differentiated human relationships and language. Rhythm first belongs to the order of the body, where heartbeat and respiration are witness to the body's vitality. From the time of birth, when placed at the mother's breast, the child associates its well-being with the familiar and comforting sound of the mother's heartbeat and the coming-and-going of her breath. This vital rhythm becomes the first signifier for a relationship to another human being for which the mother is the infant's first representative.

During this privileged time spent together, especially while breast feeding, the child or the '*in-fans*,' meaning 'unable to speak' in Latin, 'drinks' the mother's voice along with her milk, taking in both the rhythmic-musical forms of the songs and the rocking motion with his ears and kinesthetic sensations. The mother accompanies these important moments. The child simultaneously integrates natural and cultural rhythms; this transition between 'nature' and 'culture' (Schott-Billmann 2001: p.46-58) is made through the intensely nourishing, emotional relationship with the mother. If a mother puts that much heart into it, it is because she knows intuitively that she is passing on the key to the humanization process (Leroi-Gourhan 1985). This transmission happens gently. The transitional rhythm, which is imprinted upon the fetus's body, then later 'imbibed' by the infant, is also the cradle that rocks and calms the infant by containing his anxiety. At the same time, this rhythm organizes the transitional area of the mother-child experience and is a field for rhythmic games as well as a path leading toward individuation. Rhythm is also the pre-signifier that opens the way to language (Freud 1984).

2. The transitional space in Dance-Rhythm Therapy

The objective of dance-rhythm therapy is to establish solidly the capacity to differentiate, as well as other psychological and cognitive skills, in a process involving transitional rhythm. This takes place in a space for play, a transitional area where the autonomy of the patient, at first relative, can be progressively won over.

Therapy employing transitional rhythm is particularly prescribed in the treatment of psychosis, a state of generalized fusion-confusion in which 'there is no *other*'. The psychotic patient lives without any landmarks, lost in a chaotic universe where everything is fragmented, scattered and mixed up: the *other* and the self, fantasies and reality, his or her feelings which are contradictory, and the patient's ideas that are impossible for him to organize into coherent thoughts. The patient transfers ambivalent love-hate feelings onto the therapist which are difficult for both to handle. The cure involves making this symbiotic relationship evolve so that the patient can differentiate categories, distinguish the *other* by discovering alterity and overcome his generalized confusion.

This process of differentiation works along the same lines as the process engaged by the mother, where the psychological and ethical rules of respecting the dignity of the adult patient are reactivated. It would actually be inappropriate and offensive to make an adult patient do infantile and regressive activities that might increase dependency on the therapist. Judiciously, the art therapist uses artistic and cultural experience which is, according to Winnicott, the extension of the child's transitional area into the adult world. Winnicott underlines that it remains active. That, in fact, the transitional area of experience gives birth to adult creativity.

Similarly, art therapy is governed by aesthetic rules, which distinguish it from classical psychotherapies in that art plays a mediation role in the therapeutic relationship. Art therapy must meet artistic standards. Fortunately for dance-rhythm therapists, the popular art available to them espouses aesthetic laws that function both ethically and therapeutically. This is not fortuitous because popular art, besides having the therapeutic advantages it shares with other art forms, namely sublimation, is inseparable from its social, educational and curative functions.

Dance-rhythm therapists are informed by an anthropological understanding of oral culture and know the reasons for its effectiveness. They draw the necessary elements from popular culture, much like mothers do, while creatively reinterpreting them in the light of advances made in modern psychology. Of particular interest is the research conducted by such psychoanalysts as D.W. Winnicott, D.N. Stern and D. Anzieu on the importance of mother-child play to the path leading to humanization.

By combining these different contributions, dance-rhythm therapists construct a well-adapted method. Rhythm is the technique, but it also defines the relationship. In order to liberate the patient from a state of psychological fusion and confusion, dance-rhythm therapists organize a route favourable to creating relationships; rhythm occupies a principal place.

3. A relationship through resonance

The first phase of this route concentrates on establishing receptivity; the 'passivity' involved with listening precedes motor activity. In the same way as the child 'drinks' the maternal lullabies, the patient is invited to receive the therapist's music and singing through the ear and through the body.

a) Shared vibrations

Songs that 'swing' and that have an underlying regular beat, work like lullabies. The anxiety of the psychotic patient is calmed because he or she is bound, contained, unified, relaxed, safe and made to feel confident, which is the indispensable condition for establishing any therapeutic relationship.

A rhythm coming from the outside, awakens the transitional rhythm already existing in the patient from his earliest moments, making the inside world resonate with the outside world. In this way, a common vibration connects the patient to the therapist. This is not entirely different from what people experience at a rock concert when they feel their hearts beating in time with the music. Euripides, 2,500 years ago, remarked in *The Bacchae* that song 'brings hearts together.'

The patient's relationship to the therapist, created through resonance with the music, is vibratory and intangible. It is respectful of the patient's autonomy and better tolerated than physical contact, which often causes reticence in psychotic patients. The relationship established through resonance is as highly charged with emotional intensity if not more so. And what is more, it transcends any negative representation of the duo relationship as a loss of liberty for the patient. For a relationship based on resonance unites the partners to a third entity, the song, which represents the culture of the group to which both patient and therapist belong. (The songs most often used by the patient-therapist dyad are those chosen from a repertory of well-known, trans-generational music. The primary rhythm, the 'beat' and the 'swing' of these favorites, is never outdated, but persists in popular, modern forms such as rock, rap and techno.) Patient and therapist participate in and are surpassed by the cultural heritage of rhythmic popular music. By waking the vibrant memories of well-loved songs, music also links the patient to his past.

This method, so simple, so ancient, creates a strong link at the inter-personal level by uniting patient and therapist. At an intra-personal level, the resonance has a unifying effect on the different registers that constitute the individual: the body, the *other*, culture and memory.

The resonance produced by listening to music, which vibrates the space between patient and therapist, constitutes the transitional area of experience, the solid common ground upon which differentiation will be developed.

b) The call of another's voice

In what mysterious way does a song that is felt by the patient's body 'call' that individual outside of him or herself? The music offered by the therapist takes the patient out of his or her gloom and away from a state of moribund narcissism. The vibrations felt by the patient grow and soon get exteriorized. Feeling confident, the patient begins to hum with the therapist or tap to the beat or slightly swing the foot, nod the head or move his or her body.

Initially discrete, these reactions, like preludes to singing and dancing, are welcomed by the therapist with a smile, and are not forced in any way. The therapist has confidence in the emergence of what seems to be awaiting, awakening that which the patient now desires to exteriorize. The therapist knows that the patient has heard the call of the rhythm in the music.

The voice of the music is twofold, like the Roman god Janus, who has two faces: one melodic and the other rhythmic. The first transmits an emotion that causes vibrations. The second is 'felt' more than it is heard as it underlies the melody. This rhythm marks the melody with dull, regular blows like the heartbeat does the melody of the mother's voice in the intrauterine concert. In our popular music, this 'other voice' is often subdued and perceived as almost more tactile than audible on account of the emergence of its uneven surface, reliefs and accents at regular intervals. Its beat runs under the melody and awakens the rhythm imprinted on each individual from the beginning of his or her existence.

c) A gesture in common

When the patient feels safe in a succession of beats whose regularity serves as a firm support, the therapist proposes that they accompany the song by clapping in unison to the beat. The medical staff supervising are often surprised to see that most of the patients, without having learned, know how to correctly mark the beat.

When both patient and therapist clap hands in cadence, their relationship takes a joyful turn. Enthusiasm wins them over. (Enthusiasm, etymologically, means to have god within in Greek, and is the emotion that characterizes popular music and dance). Their faces clear, the emotional and rhythmic resonance increases the intensity of each clap which gains in sonority and clarity. The patient and therapist are no longer in a fusional state where the boundaries between individuals are confused, but they have not yet reached a state of intrapsychic separation. Any physical, corporal contact that may have been used is now replaced by a rhythmic relationship made when two physically separate people are playing together. The rhythm is the symbol of their playful connection, "the point in time and space of the initiation of their state of separation" (Winnicott 1971: p.97). Thanks to the rhythm this is not a radical separation, instead a form of union is made possible between partners who are distinct because they are differentiated in time and space. Rhythm is what human beings use to make time perceptible. It also allows the organization of movement in time; therefore, structures space.

The therapist solicits in the patient an aptitude that Daniel Stern (1985) calls 'attunement'. This refers to the capacity to relate to another person by adjusting intensities such as volume or the gestural energy, affects, duration, movements and the number of forms. Playing together and sharing rhythm involves being attuned; for example, one game focuses on different qualities of clapping. The therapist begins by alternating clapping intensities: hard then soft, sharp then muted, spaced out then, in quick succession, for the patient to follow. Then, the therapist attunes to what the patient proposes.

In the transitional space woven by the rhythm between the partners, the 'transitional object' is not material and stable like the child's blanket or stuffed animal which are obviously associated with characteristics of the mother. It is the gesture in common, at the same time identical and shared, that becomes the symbol for the bond that is formed, a bond that is free and joyful because it unites two distinct people.

4. A transversal structure

Adjusting reciprocally to find a common gesture is not the kind of imitation where each person melts into another. The common gesture is mediated by a third entity which allows each person to attune to the *other* without losing the rhythm which is the code of primordial play.

a) Changing sensorial channels

Next, the therapist helps the patient discover that the resonance caused by being attuned 'holds' even if one modifies the form of the gesture that marks the tempo. For example, instead of clapping hands together, one can tap other parts of the body or translate the pulsation differently, by tapping the table or by tapping one's arm. Daniel Stern gives numerous examples of such transpositions made by the infant in its construction of differentiation. He gives the following example:

> "A nine-month-old boy is sitting facing his mother. He has a rattle in his hand and is shaking it up and down with a display of interest and mild amusement. As mother watches, she begins to nod her head up and down, keeping a tight beat with her son's arm motions." (Stern 1985: p.141)

The oscillation of the mother's head and the infant's gesture take different forms but they conform to the same rhythm.

The patient is invited to play games of this type and is encouraged to attune himself, not to the form chosen by the therapist, but rather to transfer the rhythm into another sensory-motor channel of his or her choice. Both therapist and patient perform actions taking different forms while respecting the same rhythm.

b) A veiled structure

Daniel Stern attributes the ability to be attuned to another person to the existence of mental representations, abstract and amodal, which can take different paths such as auditory, visual and kinesic. In the game that we described above, the therapist and patient are attuned, not by imitating one another, but by tuning into the same rhythm. This appears to confirm Stern's hypothesis concerning the unconscious existence in the psyche of some sort of trans-modal, pre-representations or unconscious structures that certain stimulation from neighbouring structures have the ability to 'awaken' by isomorphism. In this way, the child is able to "distill and organize the abstract, global qualities of experience" (Stern 1985: p.67).

Rhythm would be this unassuming and latent scheme, across different sensorial channels – motor, visual and auditory. One can 'rhythm' a sound, a gesture, a drawing. It is the invisible structure recognized under or behind, and in spite of, the form that simultaneously reveals and veils it.

We use this aptitude, present in every human being, to support the dance-therapy work proposed to psychotic patients. By constructing a method in which the underlying rhythm, the discrete beating of the music played or sung, resonates with the rhythm buried and latent in the patient. The therapist calls and mobilizes this internal rhythmic structure.

The rhythm is the invisible law, the unconscious structure shared by the patient and the therapist by which they will be attuned to each other and lay a foundation for their relationship. They are connected because they are both linked to its pulsation.

5. Rocking: a differentiation matrix

The patient-therapist duo, facing each other, either holding hands or not, sway to the rhythm. The therapist tries to imprint (or awaken when the patient has already acquired the notion of rhythm) the rhythmic structure of rocking back-and-forth, or side-to-side and then to mobilize this coming-and-going which forms the differentiation matrix.

a) Swaying to the music

Swaying is a bipolar movement – it comes and goes between two places, from the right to the left or from the back to the front and between two temporal experiences, a time for going and a time for coming back. Swaying creates a distance between two points in space and two points in time.

The therapist must not lose sight of his objective which is to help the patient gain autonomy. The therapist makes the most of the potential for differentiation contained by these bipolar rhythms to lead the patient toward the ability to differentiate between the distinct partners making up their duo. Indeed, if the therapist's desire was narcissistic rather than orientated toward serving the patient, he would be happy to charm the patient, using seduction to keep him or her under the captivating spell of the rocking motion, effectively barring the way to individuation. Rather, by trying to lead the patient to autonomy through constructing relationships based on subjectivity, the therapist corresponds to Winnicott's "good enough mother" (Winnicott 1999: p.10). The term "good enough mother" means, in fact, that she must not be 'too' good. Loving, but not fusional – she also symbolically conveys the 'father', that is to say, she is able to make a cut or break in her own relationship to the child. In order to help the child separate from her, she offers the child the means for making distinctions between people, between things, between feelings, between imagination and reality and to do this, she uses a lot of rhythm.

If the therapist is also 'good enough', he is overjoyed to see the founding moment of the cure happen when the patient discovers a break or a gap between the 'call' and the 'response'. This break or gap is the temporal space that separates and unites the two partners. The patient begins to hear a call in the rhythm and responds to it, not at the same time and in unison with the therapist, but in a differed manner, in alternation.

First, the 'call' comes from the percussion instrument (drum or tambourine) played by the therapist or musician and is accordingly formed by this. The musician plays a brief, rhythmic sequence, simple and clear, to which the patient responds by transposing the sounds corporally and vocally, attuning to its duration, intensity and emotional quality. In this game, there must not be any confusion between what is produced by the therapist or musician, the 'call', and the patient-dancer. These respective productions alternate without overlapping, and in this 'alternation' the patient discovers alterity – there is the *other* and consequently the self, two distinct beings.

Therefore, separation occurs temporally; a limited amount of time is given to the musician (his rhythmic phrase should not be long) creating an edge to his production, a break that allows the patient's response to materialize. There is a time for each partner. Also, this separation occurs spatially; there is one space for the musician and another for the patient.

b) Alternation games

The patient-therapist exchange is organized rhythmically on the call-response model in the transitional area of experience. In this face-to-face exchange, the patient and therapist take turns, producing movements, facial expressions, gestures and vocalizations, remaining quiet and still while listening to each other.

Alternation provides a 'pattern' for making many call-response games that are analogical, such as the echo game, symmetrical or complementary. At first unconstrained, little by little the patient and therapist are inscribed in the rhythmic law established by the music. The ternary rhythms give each person 3 or 6 beats, while the binary rhythm gives 2, 4 or 8 beats. The music's law provides each one the same duration, an equal place and an identical chance for expression.

Each person in turn is a transmitter of a gesture, created before the *other*, that represents him or her and then, is a receiver of the *other's* creation. The psychotic patient, like the child who plays with his mother, creates himself at the same time as he discovers the *other*.

Conclusion

Therapy suited to treating psychotic patients helps us to understand better why rhythm was selected by evolution to convey the humanising law of differentiation across generations in every society. Rhythm is what supports the alternation that creates intermittence, breaks, and periodic retreats followed by the return – disappearance preceding re-appearance. But this intermittent eclipse is humanizing in so far as the subject, temporarily effaced and leaving a place for the *other*, does not cease to exist. On the contrary, by receiving and resonating with the *other*, the subject is enriched by what he or she hears inside himself or herself which comes from the *other*.

Since rhythm provides human beings with the key for the jubilatory creation of the subject which is born of a co-creation with the *other*, it is not surprising that the Greeks represented rhythm as Dionysos, a god having creative powers. In India, it is the god Shiva. It is also not surprising that dance, the art that renders rhythm perceptible by transposing it in space was the privileged rite for celebrations. Dance-rhythm therapists feel light and confident knowing the benefits of this creative rhythm. It brings joy and strength, even to the most debilitated and fragile individuals, like those whom therapists are called upon to help.

References

Anzieu, D. (1994) *Le Moi-Peau. Paris,* Dunod.

Didier-Weill, A. (1995) *Les Trois temps de la Loi.* Paris, Seuil.

Dolto, F. (1982) *Séminaire de psychanalyse d'enfant.* Essais tome 1. Paris, Seuil.

Freud, S. (1984) Essais de psychanalyse. Payot, Paris, 1984 (1st edition 1927), p. 51-55, in "*Au-delà du principe de plaisir*" (1920 Jenseits des Lustprinzips, Gesammelete Werke, tome XIII, pp. 3-69).

Levi- Srauss, C. (1965) *La pensée sauvage.* Paris, Plon.

Leroi-Gourhan, A. (1985) *Le Geste et la Parole.* collection Sciences d'Aujourd'hui. Paris, Albin Michel.

Nancy, J-L. (2002) *A l'écoute.* Paris, Galilée.

Quignard, P. (1996) *La haine de la musique.* Paris, Calmann-Lévy.

Schott-Billmann, F. (2001) *Le besoin de danser.* Paris, Odile Jacob.

Schott-Billmann, F. (2006) *Le Féminin et l'amour de l'Autre.* Paris, Odile Jacob.

Stern, D.N. (1985) *The Interpersonal World of the Infant: A View from Psychoanalysis and Developmental Psychology.* New York, Basic Books.

Winnicott, D.W. (1971) *Playing and Reality.* London, Tavistock Publications.

Winnicott, D.W. (1997) *De la pédiatrie à la psychanalyse.* (trans. Jeanine Lamanovitch). Paris, Payot.

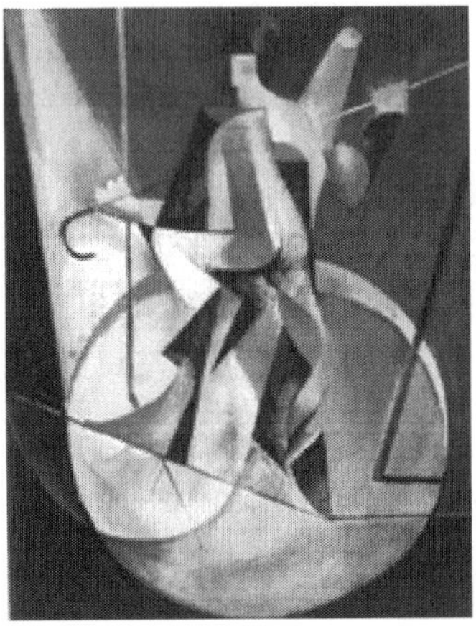

ECArTE

European Consortium for Arts Therapies Education

ECArTE is a consortium of Universities, which was founded in 1991 and currently comprises 35 member institutions from 15 European countries. It is a non profit-making organisation. Its primary purpose is to represent and encourage the development of the arts therapies at a European level, in particular courses offering nationally validated and professionally recognised education for arts therapists. (The arts therapies include art therapy, dance-movement therapy, drama therapy and music therapy.)

The Consortium's work includes:

- creating stronger European links in the arts therapies through the international exchange of staff and students
- promoting research into methods of arts therapies practice within Europe
- developing opportunities for international study in arts therapies training programmes
- promoting recognition of qualifications in the arts therapies at a European level
- supporting the development of appropriate, academically recognized, nationally validated Higher Education courses for the arts therapies
- publishing academic texts on current trends, philosophies and research in European arts therapies
- offering opportunities for professional communication at its international conferences

Hon. President
Prof. Dr. Line Kossolapow, University of Münster, Germany

ECArTE Executive Board

Chair:	Sarah Scoble, University of Worcester, United Kingdom
Vice-Chair:	Eha Rüütel, Tallinn University, Estonia
Co-ordinator:	Richard Hougham, The Central School of Speech & Drama, University of London, United Kingdom
Treasurer:	Egbert Hulshof, HAN University, Nijmegen, The Netherlands

Current Member Institutions of ECArTE

Belgium:	Arteveldehogeschool Gent Provinciale Hogeschool Limburg, Hasselt
Croatia:	Sveuciliste U Zagrebu
Estonia:	Tallinna Ülikool
Finland:	Satakunnan Ammattikorkeakoulu, Kankaanpää Jyväskylän Yliopisto
France:	Paris Descartes Université Université de Nantes
Germany:	Fachhochschule für Kunsttherapie, Nürtingen Fachhochschule für Kunsttherapie, Kunstpädagogik und Freie Kunst, Ottersberg
Ireland:	Crawford College of Art and Design, Cork
Latvia:	Riga Stradins University
The Netherlands:	Hogeschool van Arnhem en Nijmegen Christelijke Hogeschool Noord-Nederland, Leeuwarden Hogeschool Zuyd Hogeschool van Utrecht Codarts, Hogeschool voor de Kuusteu Hogeschool Leiden
Norway:	Oslo University College
Poland:	Uniwersytet WroclawskiAkademia Humanistyczno-Ekonomiczna w Łodzi
Russia:	St Petersburg Academy of Postgraduate Pedagogical Training
Slovenia:	Univerza v Ljubljani, Ljubljana
Spain:	Universidad Complutense de Madrid Universitat de Barcelona Universitat Autònoma de Barcelona (UAB)
Sweden:	Universitet, Umea Danshogskolan, Stockholm

United Kingdom: University of Hertfordshire
University of Worcester
The Central School of Speech and Drama, London
Goldsmiths, University of London
University of Derby
Roehampton University
Queen Margaret College, University of Edinburgh

BIOGRAPHICAL NOTES

JANEK DUBOWSKI

Janek qualified as an art therapist in 1977 and took up his first teaching position on the St. Albans Art Therapy training in 1980. He gained his Doctorate in Comparative Psychology in 1983. He has also completed training in counselling and then in psychotherapy and has worked both in the NHS and in private practice. Currently he holds a senior academic appointment at Roehampton University in London where he developed the first Jungian art therapy training to be offered in the UK. He was one of the founder members of ECArTE, the European Consortium for Arts Therapies Education.

VINCENT ESTELLON

Vincent is a senior lecturer at René Descartes University in Paris. A clinical psychologist, he is a member of the 'Cliniques de l'extrême' (EA 4056) team in the LPCP laboratory of René Descartes University. He works specifically on borderline behaviours. His book, *Les états limites", Que sais-je?*, was published in Paris by PUF in 2010.

DAVID READ JOHNSON

Ph.D., RDT-BCT is a founding member and former president of the National Association for Drama Therapy in the U.S, Director of the Institutes for the Arts in Psychotherapy, New York City; Co-Director of the Post Traumatic Stress Center, New Haven, Connecticut; and Associate Clinical Professor, Department of Psychiatry, Yale University School of Medicine.

CHRISTINE LAPOUJADE

PhD in Psychology. She was course co-ordinator in the Department of Arts Therapies (music-therapy, dance and drama-therapy and art therapy) at the University Paris Descartes and founder member of ECArTE. A member of the Executive Board and Chair from 2002 to 2009.

EDITH LECOURT

Edith is PhD in clinical and pathological psychology, full Professor of psychology at the University Paris Descartes. Psychoanalyst (Freudian), musician (clarinetist) and music therapist, she is a scientific referee for the training in arts therapies at her university. She was co-founder of the French Association of Music Therapy. She is author of many articles and books on music therapy, psychoanalysis and group analysis.

MARIÁN LÓPEZ FERNANDEZ CAO

Having graduated in Fine Art, Marián gained her MA in Pschycotherapeutical Interventions and her doctorate in Visual Art Education. She is currently the co-ordinator for the Masters in Art Therapy and Art Education for Social Inclusion at the University Complutense of Madrid/University Autónoma of Madrid/University of Valladolid. Marián is Director of the Institute for

Feminist Research, Director of the scientific review Arteterapia, and the author of several books in Spanish on the subjects of art as a therapy and of art and women: *Art Therapy* (2006), *Reinventing life* (2009), *Absence, memory and identity* (2011), *Recovering Memory* (1999), *Geographies of vision* (2000) and *Mulier me fecit: towards a feministanalysis on Art and Education* (2011).

MIMMU RANKANEN

Mimmu is a senior lecturer teaching art therapy in Aalto University, Department of Art since 2008 (part-time lecturer 2000-2007). She has had a private art therapy practice since 2002 for adults and adult groups. She has also been active in the field of visual art with many private and group exhibitions in galleries and museums both in Finland and internationally.

MALCOLM ROSS

Malcolm was for thirty years a lecturer in arts education at the University of Exeter, UK. Since his retirement he has continued to teach and research. He works with cultural animators at the University of Slaski in Poland and is Visiting Professor at the Institute for Integrative Arts, London Metropolitan University. His new book, *Cultivating the Arts in Education and Therapy* is this year published by Routledge. Previous publications include *The Creative Arts* (1978), *The Aesthetic Impulse* (1984), *Assessing Achievement in the Arts* (1993), and *Evaluating Education Programmes in Arts Organizations* (2002). Malcolm serves as a member of Ecarte's Publications Committee.

FRANCE SCHOTT-BILLMANN

France Schott-Billmann is a psychoanalyst, dance therapist and the Programme Leader of the Performing Arts Therapy specialisation at Paris Descartes University, France. Her research interest lies in dance and related cultural practices and she has published several books on the therapeutic function of dances and trance in traditional societies. Much in line with the work done by Katherine Dunham in the field, France Schott-Billmann's anthropological reading of these rituals informs her approach to dance therapy. Her most recent publications are *Le Besoin de Danser* (Odile Jacob, 2001), *Le Féminin et l'Amour de l'Autre* (Odile Jacob, 2006) and *Quando la Danza Guarisce* (FrancoAngeli, 2011).

SARAH SCOBLE

Sarah Scoble is the Course Leader of the MA in Dramatherapy programme at the University of Worcester and Director of the Southwest School for Dramatherapy Limited, U.K. Formerly, she was Head of the Centre for Performing Arts and Media at South Devon College, Torquay. She has been a member of the Executive Board of ECArTE and Director of ECArTE's international conferences since 1995. She has been Chair of the Consortium since 2009.

James **Roose-Evans**

James Roose-Evans argues that a true ritual creates a space in which the inner spirit is free to move. It provides a threshold, a liminal space, which calls for a crossing over into a new life. As such, it calls for a letting go of the safe, and knowing that once we have crossed over we cannot go back. It marks a transition from one mode of being to another. A true ritual is that in-between space that leads us into the inner realm of the psyche, the ground of all our being. He considers that ritual is one of the neglected forms of theatre and suggests that what is perhaps most needed in our society is to enable people to rediscover the rich roots of their own creativity and in this way restore meaning to their lives.

Martin **Cope**

This paper extends the author's previous research-based conclusions (Cope 2005, 2006) and practice-based research findings (Cope 2009). It is argued that 'dual consciousness', the dynamic balanced interplay between the reflective and the experiential, is the key human state and goal for optimizing human development. The space between client and therapist is a potential space for the development of dual consciousness that is essential for both therapeutic facilitation and client integration. The development of relational dual consciousness is further applied to the research environment and multi-agency interventions to show how human development may be maximized. Throughout the text, the poetic insight of Kahlil Gibran (1926) upon reason and passion offers literary colour to the developingarguments.

Dianne **Gammage**

In this paper Dianne identifies some of the potent healing qualities inherent in the medium of play within the context of the therapeutic relationship. She explains why, from a Buddhist perspectives, she believes that therapy work is largely psycho-spiritual in nature. She explores the Buddhist concepts of Source, Being and Conditioned Self and describes how our conditioned self in its attempts to protect, can inadvertently imprison us in repeating old patterns of behaviour that are outdated and restrictive to psychological growth and serve to create further suffering, both to ourselves and to others. She explores how play can create a gateway to our deeper being that is inherently healthy and whole and whose propensity is towards emotional openness and expansion, interconnectedness and fundamental happiness.

Malvern **Lumsden**

Focusing on the individual body in therapy can be detrimental if it lacks a focus on moving in space (including moving in relationship to other people). Moving in space is what most distinguishes dance movement therapy from other body and arts therapies. Conversely, it is the relationship to self, emotion, relationship and metaphor that most distinguishes dance movement therapy (DMT) from purely *physical activity* approaches to general and mental health. This paper explores three aspects of *space* – the external world, the internal world, and the transitional world between them, how they interact, how they impact upon the development of a Spatial Self, and their implications for therapy. The Spatial Self is seen as one of (currently twelve) facets of a Sense of Self, a facet which, in therapy, may need building up, restoring, rebuilding and integrating, not least in the context of what is being called developmental trauma disorders.

Brenda **Meldrum**

In this paper, metaphor in dramatherapy is defined as the medium of therapeutic change, giving the client safety to tell her or his story. The paper takes a developmental approach based on John Bowlby's attachment theory of relationships, tracing development through the infant's use of symbols, to sensory, projective, socio-dramatic and fantasy play into play therapy and to dramatherapy. The paper argues, with Bruce Wilshire, that theatre is a metaphor of life, as persons in "real life" act in a theatre-like way. The theatre model of dramatherapy is described and three case studies are presented as illustrations of the text.

Regine **Merz**

HIV infection is a global challenge. Worldwide there are 33.4 million people living with HIV and AIDS (UNAIDS 2009). In Europe the number of newly diagnosed infected people is increasing. The situation is dramatic in Eastern Europe. The number of infections have increased here over the last 10 years by a factor of 20. And the new diagnoses concerns people between fifteen and twenty-four years old. An end to this dramatic development is not clear yet. Dealing with a chronic lifelong illness is challenging. Regine asks, 'can art therapy satisfy the needs of people with HIV and AIDS? And if art therapy is a useful method, how can it be integrated into the treatment and provision of the HIV infection?'

Heidrun **Panhofer**

This article puts forward some of the outcomes of a recent study on the extent to which the embodied experience can be put into words. A surprising, unexpected side-result of the study showed that the applied methodological procedures may be a useful practice for clinical supervision. Of the several different models developed, two models for group supervision i.e. for large and for small groups, are presented here in a manualised version, serving as practical examples of how to access the knowledge of the body. The procedures integrate the paradigm of 'significant moments' and shift from writing to movement and then again writing, allowing one to work with the supervisees' capacity of "thinking in movement" in order to access non-languaged realms of knowing or "prenoetic" spheres. The different models of group supervision presented here are an invitation for supervisors from DMP, body psychotherapies, arts therapies, but also for any verbal therapies to investigate the connection between embodied experience and the embodied word in order to explore the intercorporeal perspective of the therapeutic relationship.

Helen **Payne**

This paper examines a pilot study of an intervention which aimed to close the gap between the psyche and the soma termed the BodyMind Approach (BMA) was systematically evaluated. It appeared to help patients suffering chronic somatic symptoms, unexplained by classifications from biomedical illness, to create meaning from movement and body-felt senses arising from their bodily symptoms. Inner worlds were explored, shrinking the distance between psyche and soma. Those with medically unexplained symptoms (MUS) – a generic term for somatoform disorder/ psychosomatic symptoms – are 10-20% of all primary care consultations, greater in secondary care, and these are chronic, heartsink patients who do not easily access psychological therapies such as CBT/counselling. The former, is only effective for those few willing to try it, and only in the short term. The intervention in this study is derived from dance movement psychotherapy and authentic movement, using the inter-relationship between body and mind within a supportive, facilitated group. Outcomes (from a mixed methodology - quantitative and qualitative) from the study, undertaken at the interface between primary community care in the UK NHS, showed increased activity levels and wellbeing; more effective coping/functioning strategies; reduction in anxiety/ depression, GP-consultation and medication usage, and symptom distress. All changes were maintained at 3-month follow-up and were supported by qualitative analysis.

Daniel **Stolfi**

Daniel explores how puppetry can be used as a dramatherapeutic medium with adult populations. He suggests the need for extensive research in order to develop further what is a neglected and under-utilized but potentially rich dramatherapy medium. The central premise of this paper is that the use of therapeutic puppetry is as applicable and valid to adults as it is with children. Given the potential overlap between the symbolic and liminal characteristics of puppetry as a sophisticated and nuanced mode of expression and the symbolically luminal spaces adults inhabit in therapeutic settings, puppetry is particularly suited to address adult issues in ways that may not be easily accessed by other routes. Daniel draws on examples from his work with adult male offenders that formed part of his recent MA dissertation and was influenced by the psychoanalytic and anthropological viewpoints of Winnicott, Van Gennep, and Turner. The idea of crossing thresholds is suggested by the confluence of these inter-related perspectives. In line with the recent ECArTE conference theme of The Space Between: the potential for change, the paper explores some of the ways therapeutic puppetry incorporates this theme of space with adults.

Mark **Wheeler**

In 2011, therapists must acknowledge that there is a cell-phone or smartphone in the pockets of most of our clients. The therapist in 2011 must remain mindful of the multidimensional implications of this tiny electronic object. Smart-phones create in the therapy room a new borderline between the outside world and the therapeutic space. Clients no longer have their world contained in their heads and a few discrete objects in their pockets or handbags. Clients may now be carrying vast databases and information resources in their pockets or bags, whether this is consciously acknowledged or not. To make conscious this new relationship with a containing object invites new triangulations for the arts therapist. What are the issues when therapists are invited to view clients' JPEG galleries and MPEG files? What are the ethical considerations? What are the iconic and talismanic properties? What is the phenomenology of these encounters? Mobile telephone photography is probably now the most widely practised outsider art in the developed world. Its practice, including immediate uploading of images onto virtual public spaces, informs us more immediately about contemporary psychological evolution than academic studies can. What does the rapid assimilation of this new technology tell us about attachment?

Latifa **Benabou Lucido**

Latifa relates her former research, on social representations, social identity, international migrations and issues of multi-disciplinarity to the arts therapist's professional identity, by exploring the professional position of working with students whilst on clinical placements. It brings up questions linked to the "space between" and to the place of the emerging arts therapies profession.

Keywords: arts-therapy, professional identity, professional position, academic training, professional associations, "l'entre-deux", the space between.

Cristina **Dias Allessandrini**

This paper discusses the potential for change presented in scientific research conducted throughout Brazil, upon different areas of knowledge, focusing on Art Therapy. Data was collected on scientific works developed by Brazilian Art Therapists in stricto sensu courses such as Masters and Doctorate programs, and Art Therapy works from students of lato sensu post-graduation courses. A database was then created, considered fundamental to the recognition of Art Therapy as a profession and aiming to enable ongoing data interchange among Brazilian Art Therapists, to explore the space between different areas and where to achieve and perform, and facilitate interdisciplinary confluence and exchange.

Rene **Lesné**

In contemporary art, the space between the work of art and the viewer has profoundly changed. Works of art exhibited in salons, then in galleries and museums, placed under the gaze of viewers, call for the latter's assessment and increasingly demand their critical attitude. This process, under the aegis of the works' value as 'exhibits', posits an autonomous space of art, an 'art world'. When placed in this 'art world', or when positioned in relation to this institutional space, works of art gradually change their character and acquire new features. Once they have become fully part of the process of arts publication, art works assume unexpected shapes; in modifying their characteristics as objects, they reinvent themselves by virtue of their place in the space (as 'installations', for example) or their occurrence (as 'happenings'). This repositioning of the work simultaneously repositions and modifies the role of the viewer.

Martine **Colignon**

Martine was invited to respond to Rene Lesné's paper, in order to explore how contemporary art can affect the arts therapist's practice. She explains how she makes a bridge between art as artistic knowledge and practice and art as a therapeutic practice; how she manages this in-between position which is so difficult to maintain and yet is precisely what constitutes art therapy.

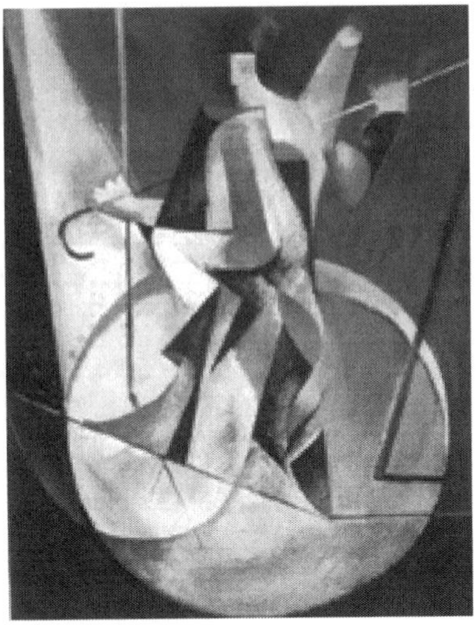

Cover picture

Tightrope Walker by Chris Hoggett, from his pictorial journal *The Joker*, reproduced by kind permission of the artist.

Chris Hoggett exhibited his work and spoke of his transformative journey through art at ECArTE's 10th European Arts Therapies Conference, in London, in 2009. Chris is a former stage designer and accomplished artist who has produced a substantial body of work over 20 years as a response to manic depression. The artwork comprises over 600 items, mainly paintings, drawings, collages, reliefs, etchings and photographs, and a small number of ceramics, stage costumes and sculptures. He has published a catalogue of the artwork, together with a commentary on each piece, under the title The Joker: Self Transformation through Art and Dream. The commentaries include interpretations of artworks in terms of Chris's struggle with manic depression and draw heavily on his dream journals.

The cover picture was developed from an earlier painting of the artist's, in which a figure is unwinding or loosening-up and stepping out of a chair. Subsequently, the chair becomes a bicycle, as the rider decides it is time to move on.

Chris Hoggett writes in his journal: "As the chair transformed itself into a vehicle and the figure pedalled away, it followed it was likely that the chair could be removed entirely. So what would happen to the figure?" The cover image was one of the artist's attempts to answer that question. "The figure is above the circus ring – one couldn't ask for more space than this – It has now become a balancing act."

How to find out more:

Enquiries and purchase requests for *The Joker*: Self Transformation through Art and Dream can be made via

email: **mike@mikehogget.co.uk**

or visit **www.chrishoggett.blogspot.com**